Rescuing Ourselves from Chemtrails, Clots and Cancers

Wendy Daniel

Rescuing Ourselves from Chemtrails, Clots and Cancers

ISBN: 978-1-923631-03-8 (paperback)

Published in Australia by Wendy Daniel.
Printed in Australia by InHouse Publishing, Print & Design.

INHOUSE PTY LTD PUBLISHING

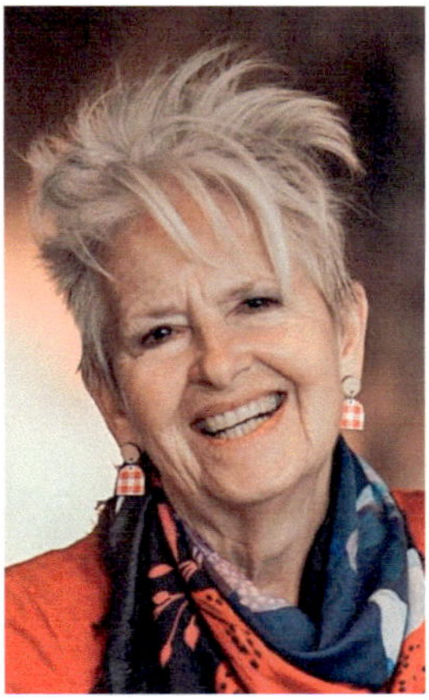

Dear Readers,

Who am I and how do I come to be writing a book like this?

I have no medical background, which is a huge advantage in these strange times. I can write as I see fit, moving seamlessly in this particular book between the factual, the possible, the anecdotal and the intuitive without risking a career, a job, an income, a reputation, or even a colleague's nod of approval.

I started researching vaccines when my first grandchild was born over sixteen years ago. I was puzzled by the lack of real information or statistics in the leaflets at the doctor's office and soon realised that all the independent research and statistics actually pointed to vaccines being harmful. Virtually every statement in my first book: Vaccines, Myths and Facts, now in its fourth edition, is backed up by original, independent studies, facts and quotes. These prove that vaccines have undergone startlingly little official testing and cause significant harm on a regular basis. It's a clear and simple warning about their use.

The second book: 'Detox after Covid and Thrive', was written with the amazing support of four Australian naturopaths. If you trusted your medical doctor in the pre-covid era, are suffering after the shots or are new to detoxing and eating clean, I encourage you to read Detox after Covid and Thrive first, before you start on this book. It's more of an instruction book summarising what many wonderful researchers and healers had discovered at the time about recovering after covid and the experimental jabs. It includes some of the basic principles of taking responsibility for your own health, including how to choose a good practitioner.

People who had once been compliant with the mainstream and were suffering the consequences finally had a simple road map to help them find their own way back to health. It's part of the story and a really good start but, as it turns out, not the whole story in the post-covid era.

I thought after Detox after Covid and Thrive, that my work on detoxing in these strange times was done. I'd listed nine good websites which seemed to be at the leading edge of Covid research around the world. I had led interested readers over to them and I believed these sites would continue giving people ongoing updates as the situation unfolded. All seemed to be well.

Then a young and gifted psychic told me out of the blue during lunch with friends that I had another book to write on detoxing.

Seriously? I thought I was done …?

She was right.

That's exactly the way it turned out. It often seems that if you're going to write about something, whether its detoxing or divorce, eventually you'll have to experience it yourself.

So here we are ….

The book in your hands is much closer to the leading edge. Where is the leading edge anyway? Is it a small step, or a cliff edge? We don't know. It's one of the many things we don't know. This book starts as a mainly personal journey beginning with a single slide on a dark field microscope and progresses through virtually unchartered territory like an early explorer hacking through thick bushland.

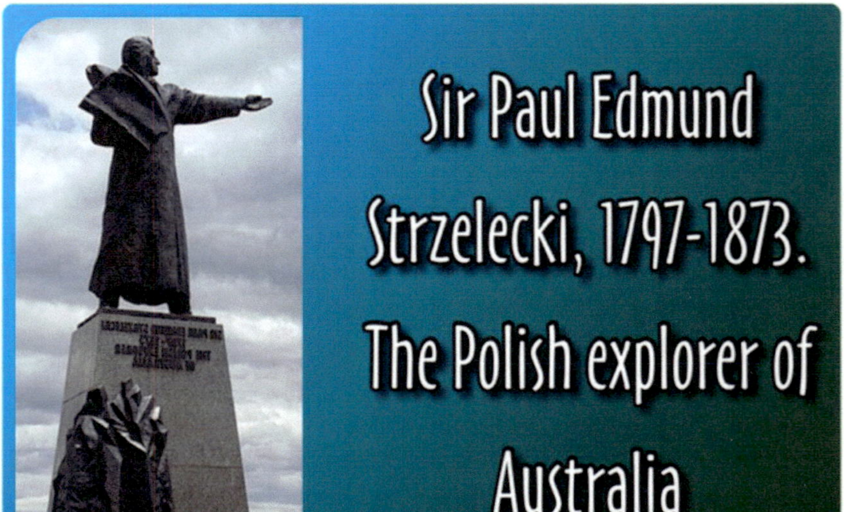

I wish with all my heart that I could soften the blow, but I don't think I can. We have to rip off the band-aid …

There's the bad news and the good news …

The bad news:

The vast majority of us in the developed world (vaccinated and vaccine-free alike) have been contaminated and it's worse than we thought. The main aspects of it all are:

- Nano-filaments assembling in our blood, making us more vulnerable to electro-magnetic frequencies.
- Genetically modified pathogens.
- A wide range of manufactured snake and snail venoms
- Parasites of many shapes, sizes and habits that we know to check for in our animals but not in ourselves.
- Universities and research institutions are not interested.
- The vast majority of doctors can't help.
- We still have many more questions than answers.

One thing is certain: The general quality of our blood in the western world has deteriorated since 2022.

Even if we're in good shape, I believe that if we want to thrive in the world today, we need to pay much closer attention to the state of our blood. I am not alone in this belief.

It's possible that if we ignore it, this new contamination may accumulate, stealing our energy and oxygen, blocking our vital systems and making us more susceptible to a host of other onslaughts in the body including reproductive issues, respiratory infections, circulation issues and turbo cancers.

The good news:

A few dedicated, self-funded people around the world have not only identified these mysterious manufactured anomalies but seem to have discovered some effective ways to keep them under control.

Once I realised this and started to write, I was picking up scattered clues and statements like little nuggets of truth in thick bushland from the few dedicated practitioners and researchers actually brave enough to speak about them. Sometimes people were prepared to be named. Sometimes they weren't. Sometimes the clues fitted together. Sometimes they didn't. Sometimes the scientists agreed with each other. Sometimes they didn't. Sometimes they even called each other names. Sometimes scientists acknowledged there was an issue. Sometimes they didn't. Sometimes they seemed to be talking about completely different issues. Sometimes it seemed that what I was listening to was a deliberate muddying of the waters.

I believe that no-one has described the situation we are facing more accurately or concisely than a woman who usually prefers to be known as Nomoresilence. All links are live on my website https://www.lightoftruths.net/ and I invite you to listen to this short clip:

http://rumble.com/v72vt20--reclaim-our-terrain-.html

Nomoresilence talks about what is happening to our blood and how we can overcome it: https://rumble.com/v72vt20--reclaim-our-terrain-.html

I hope you will choose to join me on our expedition into this unmapped territory and use your own skills, experience and common sense to make what you can of the clues we find along the way. It gives me no pleasure whatsoever to be the bearer of bad news. I wish I was wrong, but it's no exaggeration to say that our lives may depend on it.

Since 2021, I've documented something unprecedented under my microscope in live blood analysis, structures and behaviours never seen before in living human blood. These changes in the blood are universal, regardless of geography, vaccine status or health.

The calamari clots are still seen in our EBOO lines and the embalmers' findings. They are not transient. They self-assemble and are responsive to frequency.

I do not believe that what I am seeing is random. These structures are real, consistent, synthetic in nature and part of a deliberate process.

I believe they are delivered via multiple routes, the jab, food, water, air, dental anaesthetics, environment, chemtrails and energetic programming.

I believe this is a quiet, deliberate alteration of the human terrain, biologically, neurologically and spiritually. We need to find the courage to speak out about this.

I still believe we have the solutions. In my opinion these anomalies are just pollution. We can detoxify the body and break these structures down.

It's time to step up, tell the truth and reclaim what was always ours. Our right to be whole, free and human again.

Summarised and adapted from Nomoresilence https://rumble.com/v72vt20--reclaim-our-terrain-.html

My aims with this book are:

Firstly: That we everyday human beings can understand some of the basics of this threat and find some ideas and suggestions in these pages that we can use to protect ourselves safely.

Secondly: That open minded naturopaths, doctors, scientists, researchers or anyone with an alert mind, an open heart and a bit of time will be able to use some of the ideas and starter points in the references and begin their own research to head off this threat. We need all the help we can get.

I have tried to steer a path between creating needless fear and lulling us all into a false sense of security.

We have to rescue ourselves . . .

There are no guarantees on this important expedition. Like the explorer, Strzelecki, we are pressing forward through the bush, building our own path as we go.

Heavy though this subject is, I've tried to make it as accurate, light, simple and easy to read as I can.

Love and Light,
Courage and Truth
Wendy Daniel
June 2026

PS. I had a wonderful childhood. Not perfect by any means but blessed in so many ways.

Asking my mother about it many years later she just said 'We did the best we could at the time.'

I'm deeply grateful for that.

It's all anyone can ask for.

I stand on the shoulders of giants again with this book. It's not perfect by any means, but I did the best I could at the time.

I want to put in a
disclaimer up front that I am
not a medical practitioner, nor
a microscopist and
absolutely none of this is
medical advice.
I write from my own
experience and very basic
research for the good of all
but as at
June 2026, this is a new,
confusing and rapidly
developing situation.
I encourage you to consider
teaming up with a truly open-
minded health professional
who is willing to partner with
you on this journey.
This information is,
as they say,
for
entertainment purposes
only.

I also want to make it very clear here that I haven't taken any commission from any of the businesses I mention or recommend.
I have been very specific in recommending particular brands and practitioners in good faith where I can.
In this rapidly developing situation, it's important that you have quick access to quality products, information and contacts.
I'm doing my best, but there are no guarantees here either.

I come from an era when it was completely unthinkable for pregnant women who wanted the best for their babies to smoke, drink alcohol, take a vaccine or a pill unless absolutely essential.

Many of the ideas and suggestions here may not be safe for pregnant women.

Use your common sense and consult a natural practitioner for guidance.

Lexicon

As we navigate this unchartered territory and take control of our own health there are many new words, remedies and concepts for us to get our heads around. When we're taking in a new concept, the more words we don't understand the more likely we are to lose interest and leave it in the too-hard-basket. It's like learning a new language. It's also easy to use words we've picked up along the way without really understanding what they mean, or which now have slightly different meanings, so there are some familiar terms in here as well.

The handful of doctors and scientists talking at the leading edge of this try to stay with basic language, but have a tendency to slip into science mode and lose everyday people. What's more, the field is so new that different researchers use different words for the same microscopic findings. I've been shocked at how many new words there are. I'm adding a handy lexicon to outline some of the main words.

So we only have one list to navigate as we rescue ourselves, I have also included some supplements that may be useful for us on the way. These are marked with an asterisk *. I've tried to make it as accurate and simple as I can, but there are no guarantees.

It's quite a list! You don't need to understand - or even read it - right now. It's just here waiting for you if you come across unfamiliar words as you explore this new territory. It's a bit like looking at a map before you set out. You might like to scan it quickly before we pull on our big boots, pick up our compass, and venture into the unmapped bush together, starting our search at page 51 …

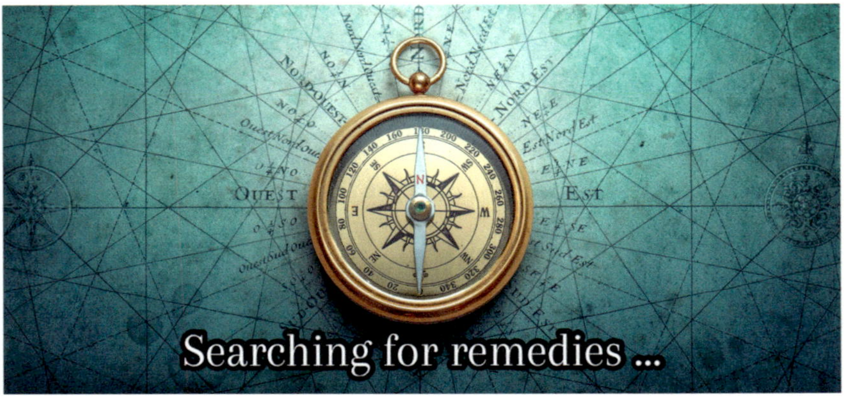

Aerobic: Improving oxygen levels, often with exercise, to encourage deep breathing and increased circulation.

Anaerobic: Living or active without free oxygen. Bacteria, fungi, moulds, parasites and other nasties like to live in low-oxygen areas in the body and the environment.

Acetylcholine: This acts as a chemical messenger, sending signals between different parts of the body and the brain. Our cells have nicotinic-acetylcholine receptors on their surface which respond to these substances.

*Activated Charcoal: This is a very porous form of carbon which binds to heavy metals like lead, mercury and cadmium in the digestive tract. It doesn't remove these metals from the tissues but picks them up and escorts them safely out of the body once they are dislodged. It plays an important part in the detox process.

Aluminium: A metal mined from deep underground which is great for aeroplanes and appliances. Despite the fact that it's used in many vaccines and is regularly found in chemtrails, it has no place in the human body.

Amyloid: A waxy, translucent fibrous protein cluster usually associated with Alzheimer's disease which, when misfolded, can accumulate in the brain, heart, or kidneys and, more recently, the veins and arteries. These misfolded proteins can disrupt normal tissue functions.

Amyloidosis: 'This is a blood-borne systemic protein misfolding disorder. It was rare in the pre-covid era but since the covid shots, it's common. We might think of amyloidosis as if someone put a jar of peanut butter into the petrol tank of our car or turned our blood into the consistency of lumpy custard.

Anti-Oxidant: reduces inflammation in the body.
/Free-radical: creates inflammation and stress in the body.
I've heard a speaker describe anti-oxidants and free radicals memorably like a dis-functional couple in a household. The free radical molecule is like the partner who always creates havoc around the house, plays loud music, upsets the neighbours. Makes a

mess all over the place, gives the kids ice-cream for dinner and lets them watch tv until the early hours. The anti-oxidant is like the partner who tidies up and fixes everything, washes up, makes peace with the neighbours, does the laundry, makes a healthy dinner, calms everyone down, baths the kids, puts them to bed and restores order.

Apoptosis: This is when a portion of your cells 'decide' to die because they are old or diseased. A bit like autumn leaves on the trees, they sacrifice themselves in order to make way for fresh new cells and healthy growth.

Artefact: Something you observe (maybe under the microscope) which looks real but which is actually created by your methods rather than by nature.

ATP: adenosine triphosphate. The major source of energy for cellular reactions and the human body as a whole. It is produced by the mitochondria.

Autophagy: This is linked to apoptosis and cell death. When we eat less, the body has to find, clean up and absorb old cells to make healthy new ones and the leaner and healthier we become.

Barium: Although it is occasionally used to create contrast in medical imaging, barium is potentially toxic to the human body.

*Bee Pollen: This is a complete protein source which also has B vitamins, iron and zinc.

*Berberine: This is an ancient medicine also found in turmeric. It may be helpful with gut health, heart problems and obesity.

Bio-engineering: How the man-made world is set up to alter our human bodies … not always for our benefit.

Bio-medical doctor: A doctor who studies the root cause of illness and the methods for curing it with both natural and pharmaceutical methods.

*Black Salve: This is a powerful and controversial salve which I have used successfully several times on skin cancers. It draws impurities and cancers near the surface out of the body into a scab-like eschar. As a natural mixture, black salve cannot be patented, this means that pharmaceutical companies and the medical system prefer to demonise it.

*Calcium Disodium EDTA. This is the type of chelation which is used to remove toxic metals and minerals from the tissues ready to be flushed out of the body as quickly as possible. It can be taken by mouth and is relatively gentle on the body. It also takes out good metals and minerals like magnesium, calcium, iron and zinc and so it's important to replace these minerals after taking it.

Cannula: This is a hollow tube which is injected into the bloodstream and held in place with a special band-aid. It allows blood to be drawn or medication, nutrition or blood therapies to be delivered into the bloodstream.

Calamari (or rubbery) clots: Not widely seen until 2022, just after the covid shots were rolled out, these are very tough clots with a rubbery, calamari-like texture.

A large study of U.S. embalming businesses in 2025, found rubbery clots in 20-30% of veins and arteries of the deceased. Clifford Carnicon and Dr Ana Milhacea tell us that the clots are made of polyamides, polyethylene and vinyl plastic polymers. Nickel, and silicon have also been found.

According to Clifford Carnicon, Dr Ana Milhacea and Dr Ed Group, they are linked to the contents of some covid shots and chemtrails. These are also seen in the living. They may be worse in the vaccinated and can cause strokes and heart attacks.

In extreme cases these clots can usually be cleared out with EBOO (Extra Corporeal Blood Oxygenation and Ozonation), EDTA interventions and special laser treatments.

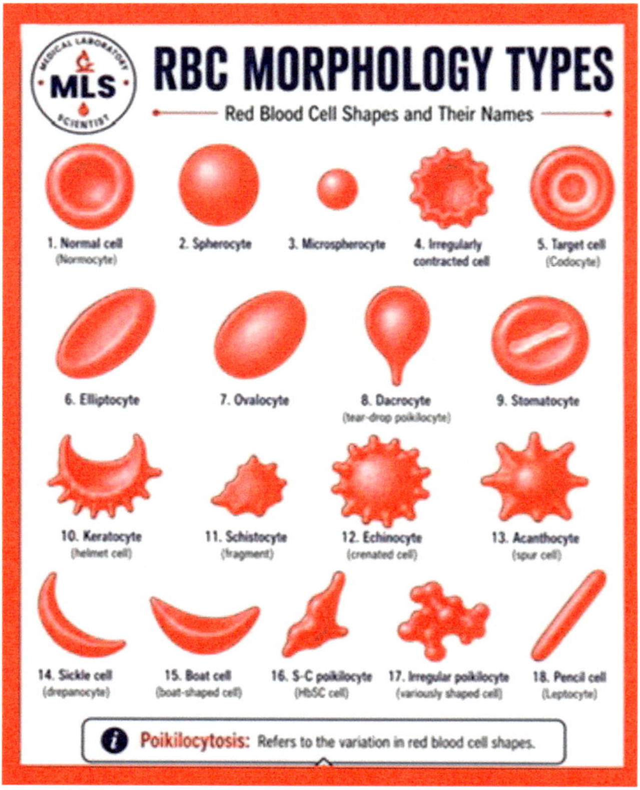

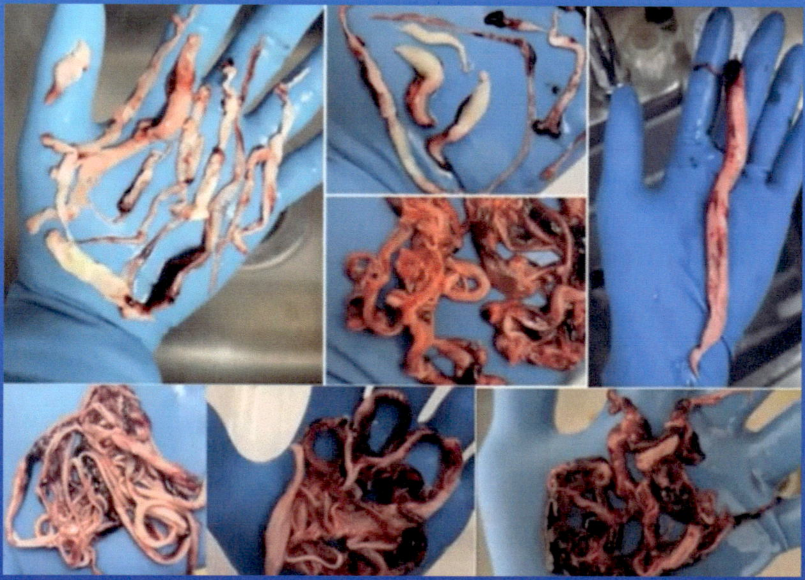

White rubbery clots being found globally by embalmers are real - not rare.

Cells: Red blood cells or Erythrocytes: One of the smallest living organs in the body. There are about 5 million red blood cells in a single drop of blood. They live for three to four months. Red blood cells don't have many mitochondria but are crucial for transporting haemoglobin and oxygen around the body.

Cells: White blood cells or Leukocytes: There are about 10 thousand white blood cells in a single drop of blood. If you have a low white blood count you may be more susceptible to infections.
They are cells of the immune system and help protect the body against infections, bacteria, fungi, parasites and (if they are strong and plentiful enough) shiny ribbons of self-assembling nano-filament fairy lights.

Chelation: This is the removal of heavy and toxic metals such as aluminium, lead or mercury from the blood either using formulations taken by mouth or intravenously in the clinic. Chelation can also strip the body of good metals so beneficial minerals like iron and zinc may need to be replaced.

Chemtrails: Part of the geoengineering program. These are trails from special high-altitude aeroplanes. They seem to fly from secret airfields and don't appear to be regulated by any visible or accountable government bodies. Their pilots are often the mercenaries of the aeronautical world. The chemtrails form huge lines of clouds which spread out and block out the sun and they are made of random selections of toxic particles: aluminium, barium, strontium, cesium, metallic salts, moulds, nano-filaments and other chemicals. All of these can disrupt normal bodily absorption and processes. (Clifford Carnicom, the Carnicom Institute)

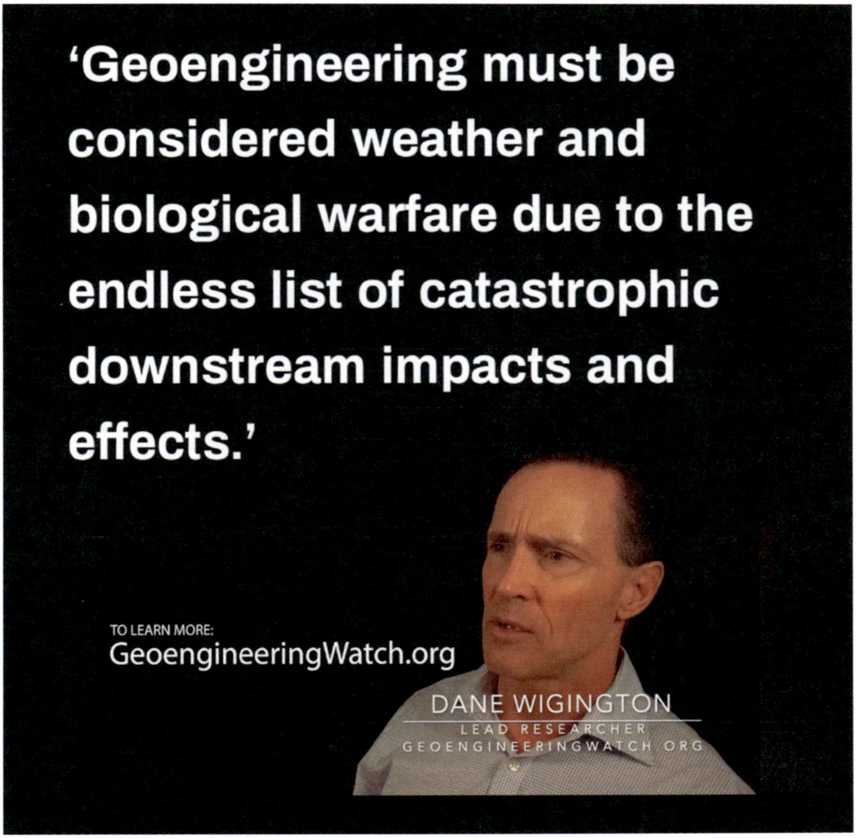

Chimera: In this subject, a chimera is a pathogen with genetic material from two or more other types of disease producing organisms. It can be natural or created in a lab.

*Chlorine Dioxide Solution (CDS): Primarily used as a water purifier. When used correctly, this is relatively gentle on the stomach and very useful as a blood purifier to help clear many parasites including malaria.

*/Magic Mineral Solution (MMS) This is closely related to CDS but often better for use diluted in a spray bottle on the skin.

Coherence: Coherence can apply to sound, light or frequency.
We might think of it like a good choir singing in harmony. We can understand the words and the message flows with beauty and clarity. Our bodies understand and respond to coherent frequencies.

/Incoherence: Incoherence is a bit like a big group of children all shouting different things at you all at once. We can't understand any of them and the whole experience is frustrating to all concerned. This description might often apply to our modern world.

Conspiracy theory: A phrase used to deliberately ridicule people who think critically, question and research what they are being told.

Contagion: This is a controversial word in today's world. Some doctors say it's a myth. While there may be many causes, every one of us has a lived experience of infection sweeping through a kindergarten, a classroom, a workplace or family. Many of these infections give us life-long immunity afterwards.

Covid shots: These varied wildly from batch to batch. None of them were beneficial but I hold the faith (optimistically) that many of them may have been saline. The quality control of any jab or vaccine is appalling and we have no idea exactly what went into individual arms.

Cross-domain bacteria: These are small species of bacteria which reproduce but which have artificial elements. (Clifford Carnicon)

*Curcumin: The main active ingredient of turmeric, it is an anti-oxidant which helps fight inflammation and promotes heart and brain health. Combining Turmeric with black pepper increases absorption of curcumin enormously.

*D3 Vitamin: This is a very important nutrient and I believe many people should be supplementing with it, especially during the winter months.

Dark Field Microscopy: Many substances can be studied with dark field microscopy but in the context of live blood analysis, a tiny drop of live blood from your finger is taken carefully and examined on a slide against a dark background to see the health of the living cells and the surrounding blood plasma.

DARPA: Defence Advance Research Projects Agency: A dark and secretive government agency. It is widely known that their technology is decades ahead of what the public is allowed to know about. The word 'defence' is often used within these agency documents when the word 'attack' might be more appropriate.

D-Dimer test: Little used before 2022, An elevated D-Dimer test measures if clots within the human body are being broken down properly by the body's own 'plasmin' or prescription drugs like Heparin, Warfarin or Cumadin. It doesn't tell you what is causing the clots.

Dental Anaesthetics: Starting around 2022, Ana Milhacea and a small international group were concerned to see nano-micro-structures assembling in insulin and dental anaesthetics, as well as many of the covid shots. In a sane world these would have been identified by medical and dentistry authorities and stopped within a week or two. They are still common. Microscopists are still finding these filaments in dental anaesthetics and usually recommend that people detox after having dental work done. These anaesthetics can be made much safer using Tri-vortex technology, as mentioned in the links.

Dialysis: A medical procedure which removes waste and extra fluids from the blood when the kidneys can't manage to do it themselves.

*DMSA: (Dimer-capto-succinic Acid) This is a chelating agent used to remove heavy lead toxicity from the body.

*DMSO: (Dimethyl sulfoxide) An off-patent medication or cream which penetrates the skin and membranes easily and can help with muscle and joint pain. As one writer puts it, 'DMSO doesn't just heal, it delivers anything you pair it with straight into your cells.'

DNA (Deoxyribo-Nucleic Acid): This is the molecule that carries the genetic instructions used in the growth, development, functioning, and reproduction of all known living organisms. It contains the complete set of information needed to build and maintain an organism and is often called the 'blueprint of life'.

Dual-Filtration Plasma Apheresis. This is lesser-known name for a closed-circuit form of dialysis intended to clear clots from the veins and arteries.

EBOO (Extra Corporeal Blood Oxygenation and Ozonation)

This must be done in a certified clinic. It's done recently because the veins and arteries are overwhelmed with various clots. It's a form of dialysis in which the blood is drawn from one vein, sent through a filter, which removes all manner of blood clots, natural and artificial nasties which may be lurking in the blood. The blood is then boosted with ozone to oxygenate it before it's put back into the body through another vein.

It takes less than an hour. Because our external world is so contaminated, three treatments over three weeks are recommended. As we are potentially being re-infected constantly, follow-up sessions or ongoing detox maintenance is recommended.

EDTA: (Ethylene-Diamine-Tetra-Acetic-acid). This is an acid that sticks to heavy and toxic metals, graphene and hydrogel in the blood. It then removes them from the body in a process called chelation. It can be taken in the form of drops, put into capsules or intravenously.

Intravenous EDTA: This removes heavy metals and other toxins from the veins and arteries in the clinic with a procedure that looks a bit like dialysis. EDTA can remove good minerals as well as bad ones so great care must be taken to replenish these later the same day.

Electrons: Miniscule parcels of energy with a negative charge. Electrons in haemoglobin bring life-giving oxygen to cells around the body.

Electron donors: Sunshine, walking barefoot on the beach or in open countryside, contact with trees, pets and moving water. Vitamin C and methylene blue are also electron donors.

Electron stealers are emotional baggage, pesticides, processed foods, stagnant water, toxins and air pollution.

Electron Transport Chain: This is like a little conveyor belt in the mitochondria as electrons bring energy to the cells.

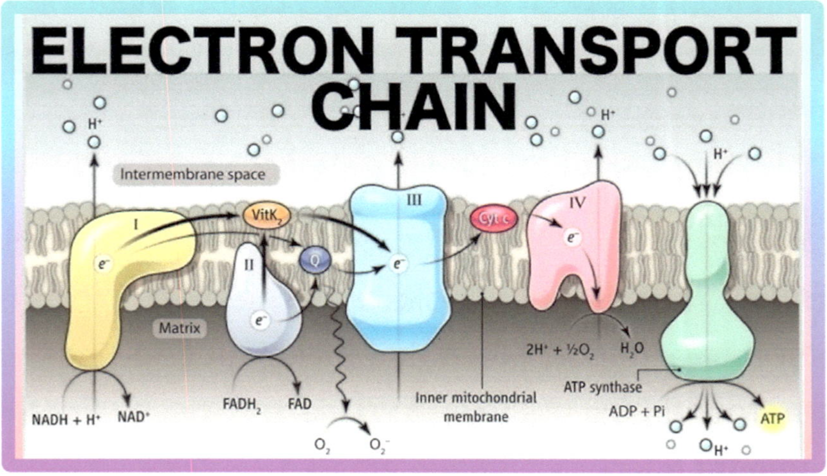

Electro smog: The electro-magnetic radiation emitted by our phones, ear pieces, microwave ovens, computers, televisions and modern appliances.

ELFET/Tri-vortex green laser (Electrical Field Entrainment Techniques.) This is a chemical-free, bio-mimicry-based process that imparts naturally optimized resonances into materials. It copies the way nature does things really well and adds vibrations to increase their effects.

EMFs (Electro Magnetic Frequencies) Many of us took our microwave ovens out of our kitchens and no longer hold our phones close to our head because we can feel for ourselves that Electro Magnetic Frequencies can be damaging. Some people are much more sensitive to this than others. Orgonite, shungite, Tachyon discs and other blocking systems and wearable pendants may help to protect you or neutralize EMF harms.

Embalming: Only about 5% of dead bodies are embalmed in Australia. In the USA and Great Britain, it's around 50%. This is a process done by funeral directors and embalmers to preserve the looks of a body so it can be viewed by friends and loved ones after death. Embalmers flush out the blood from the whole circulatory system and replace it with formaldehyde based embalming fluid. It's usually done quite easily with a single injection into the neck of the deceased. Since 2022, rubbery clots often make this impossible, even in newly deceased bodies. Many more cuts need to be done and huge clots sometimes have to be physically pulled out from limbs where they were blocking both veins and arteries.

Enema: An enema is a procedure you can do yourself with the aid of an enema bag from the chemist to help flush out toxins from the lower colon. Colonic hydrotherapy is a much deeper and more thorough cleanse.

*Enzymes: These help to speed up chemical reactions in the body such as digestion, metabolism and cellular processes.

*Essential Oils: Ana Milhacea mentions several essential oils as being useful and I have outlined these along with her other suggestions later in the book.

Expired medical patent: Pharmaceutical companies love their patents. This is how they make their big profits. Once the patent of a medication has expired, pharmaceutical companies have very little interest in it. No matter how safe or useful it might be, it becomes an unwanted orphan. This is good news for the rest of us because other manufacturers can produce it relatively cheaply. The downside is that there are no financial incentives for companies to do much needed human trials on potentially useful basic medicines and remedies.

*Fenbendazole: This is a veterinary anti-parasitic almost identical to Mebendazol which is FDA approved for humans and has an excellent safety profile. Dr William Makis and many others are getting good results by combining these into protocols which have been found to help with turbo cancers.

Fibrin: This is insoluble protein fibres in the blood. In its natural form *it looks like nice, slippery spaghetti with olive oil.* When you have a cut, it's the fibrin which quickly forms a foundational network or scaffold for the blood cells to settle and grow into before being reabsorbed as the cut heals. If fibrin comes into contact with unwanted proteins *it looks like spaghetti with a lot of parmesan cheese.* It's sticky, it's not slippery any more and can misfold, turning into a tangled mass which the body can't process. This appears to form the basis for the white fibrous clots.

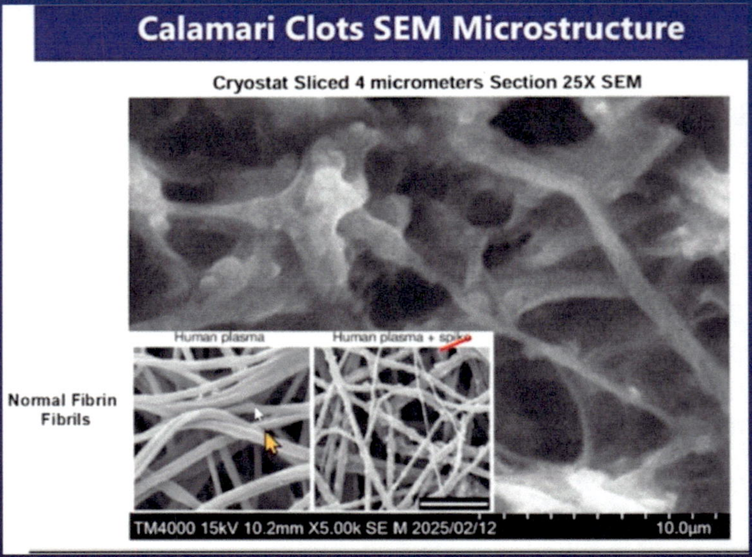

Healthy fibrin in human plasma on the left.
Human plasma and spike on the right.

Fibrinogen: This is a protein in blood plasma which mixes with thrombin and makes fibrin. This leads to normal clotting and wound healing. Since late 2022 and the roll out of covid shots this normal process seems to have been disrupted. Scientists and embalmers are still seeing tough, white rubbery clots forming in both veins and arteries.

Fulvic Acid / Humic acid: These substances are made by micro-organisms in the soil. They have been working for thousands of years improving soil nutrient absorption and detox of of heavy metals. Best bought in powder form, they are powerful for detoxification, gut health and immunity.

Gain-of-function: A term used for the practice of deliberately making a particular illness, virus or poison even more harmful to humanity. It would be nice to think of this as a diabolical conspiracy theory but, unfortunately, it's real, takes many forms and has been with us for many decades.

Glutathione: This is a powerful anti-oxidant made in the liver which helps with immune function, insulin resistance, cell health and inflammation.

GMOs (genetically modified organisms) foods and other living things which have been altered in a lab to change them in ways which our bodies don't necessarily recognise and may not be able to process.

Genetically weaponised bacteria and yeasts: It's hard to believe that companies actually do this, but they do. Dr Ed Group tells us that many bioweapons are created on brewer's yeast.

Geoengineering: Artificial weather manipulation, usually with chemtrails or frequencies.

Graphene Oxide: An experimental modified nano sized form of graphene which is so tiny it can enter the bloodstream and the cells, causing inflammation or clotting. It may interact, move and grow rapidly in the presence of EMFs and wi-fi signals.

Grounding: Connecting with nature by swimming in the sea or a natural lake, walking barefoot on the beach or grass and even touching a tree to help our bodies receive and exchange the energy we need from the earth to survive and thrive. It seems that when we exchange molecules with the living earth or waters, we are both nourished in some way.

HAARP: High-frequency Active Auroral Research Program.
This is one of the most powerful tools of weather manipulation and atmospheric control. HAARP affects cloud and storm patterns using huge numbers of antenna.
Combined with chemtrails, this is the delivery system for global weather modification.

Heparin: a drug used during EBOO treatments to thin the blood and remove any remaining clots.

Homeopathy: A system for treating disease with minute doses of substances which, if used in larger amounts, would produce the same symptoms as the disease itself. It's the energy of the substance that is used and like cures like. It can be very effective for detoxing and many other issues.

HOCATT: Hyperthermic Ozone Carbonic Acid Transdermal Technology. This is a treatment that combines steam, ozone, and carbonic acid to promote health and wellness. It aims to improve circulation, boost the immune system, detoxify the body, and boost overall vitality through a series of therapeutic modalities during a session in a specialized sauna.

Hyperbaric Oxygen therapy; A medical treatment in which healing oxygen is pumped into a chamber so it goes into the cells under pressure. I have heard anecdotal reports from a live blood analyst that if done regularly, this is useful to help the body clear most nano-technology.

Hydrogels: These structures are new in the blood since around 2022. They are a network of abnormal glowing polymers that can hold a lot of water. (We might think of them a bit like hair gel, the last thing we want gumming up our veins and arteries.) They grow and multiply on their own using the fluid in our blood, and seem to appear as self-assembling shiny micro-ribbons and pools in the blood. They can act as an antenna in the human body.

*Hydrogen peroxide: increases vital oxygen in the body. It is often used to clean cuts and grazes.

*Iodine: It's easy to find ourselves deficient in this important nutrient. It helps to regulate metabolism and protect against EMFs.

Infra-red-light therapy: (Far Infrared) This is absorbed mostly in the top layer of skin. It creates gentle heat which improves blood flow, relaxes muscles and helps relieve pain and stiffness through warming.

Infra-red-light therapy (Near Infrared): This penetrates deeper - about 1 to 5 centimetres into the body. It reaches muscles and joints, reducing inflammation, speeding wound repair and easing pain.

In vitro: In the petri dish or the glass microscope slide. Scientific experiments have to start somewhere and it's here where a lot of discoveries are made and remedies are first tested out. If they work in the lab, they might just work in the body.

In vivo: In the body. This is the real test of how a treatment works or doesn't work in practice.

Ion: An atom or molecule with an electrical charge due to gaining or losing electrons. It can be useful, as in air purifiers, but it can impact climate and health by altering the behaviour of molecules which interact with pollutants in the air.

*Ivermectin: A substance from the earth first discovered in the late 1970s and developed and patented for human use in 1987. Ivermectin has been used safely world-wide as a routine anti-parasitic medication for nearly 40 years. The people who discovered it were awarded a Nobel prize in 2015. It is currently being used with great success for treating the new turbo cancers … more on this later. Dose according to your body weight.
Some people say that due to its life-saving properties, some Ivermectin may have been adulterated in recent months and the formulation weakened by the manufacturers. For this reason, it's best to buy it from the most reputable supplier you can find.

Kinesiology: The expert use of muscle testing to connect with the higher self and reveal what the body knows. Among other things, the body will usually reveal what it needs to heal itself.

*Licorice root: This is an anti-oxidant, anti-inflammatory and anti-microbial. It's also delicious in a tea brewed with fresh ginger and lemon juice. A great, cleansing start to the day.

Liposomal: A delivery system for supplements where active ingredients are wrapped in little fat bubbles called liposomes.
This protects them from the stomach acid and allows them to be absorbed into the intestines making them more available for the body to use.

Live Blood Analysis: This is when living blood is examined under the microscope using dark field microscopy or phase contrast microscopy

*Lobelia, (Indian Tobacco): May help to treat asthma and breathing issues by relaxing the airways. It is said to help against addictions.

Long Covid: Lingering ill health from either covid or (more likely) the shots in the post covid era.

Long-Haulers: Unfortunate long-term sufferers in the post covid era.

Lyme Disease: Lyme disease is a group of many tick-borne diseases and was first described in the seventies. It's one of those strange new illnesses which your doctor may tell you is in your imagination but which is said to have been made more harmful in a lab. Lyme lives in the cells and symptoms vary widely. They include chronic fatigue, inflammation and brain fog and they can sometimes be cleared using Chlorine Dioxide (CDS) used as soon as possible. General improvements in health and liver function are always helpful.

Robert F Kennedy Jr interviews Kris Newby author of 'Bitten', The back story of Bioweapons & Lyme Disease

https://rumble.com/v48ge19-rfk-jr.-interviews-kris-newby-the-terrible-truly-awful-backstory-of-bioweap.html

Mesogen: According to an experienced EBOO microscopist, mesogens are large non biological synthetic structures which are found in the live blood of many patients They act as a conductor so they are a central command hub within the body's terrain. They cluster and self-assemble. They can disrupt the blood flow in the body and they respond to outside frequencies. They look like clustered jewellery.

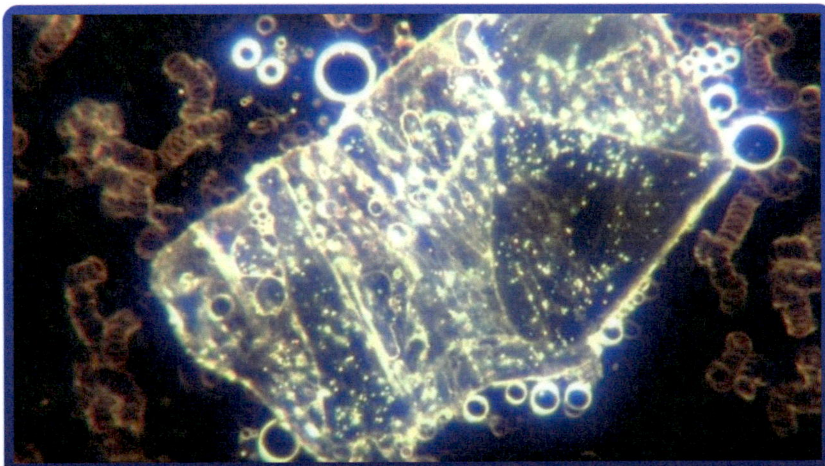

From 'Overcoming the Global Depopulation Agenda.' Dr Ana Milhacea: COVID 19 unvaccinated blood - self-assembling mesogen microchip. Magnification 2000x.

Metabolic: The organic functions in a cell, an organism or a body that are necessary for life.

Methylation: This is the process affecting the regulation of cell processes, including embryo development, detoxing, cancer and ageing.

Methylene-blue: The blue dye which was first used in hospitals to bring oxygen and life back to patients hanging in the balance on the operating table. It is being rediscovered as a powerful energiser bringing oxygen and electrons to the cells. For a substance that has so much healing potential, it has attracted more than its fair share of controversy and critics.

Micro or micron: This is a measurement: One millionth of a meter. This is about the size of a bacterium. A human red blood cell is 7-8 microns in diameter. Much of the new contamination in our blood is larger than a nanometer but smaller than a micron.

Mitochondria: The powerhouses of the cells responsible for creating energy in the body. Cells with the most mitochondria are the heart, brain and muscles. They may have 5-10,000 mitochondria per cell.
Cells with the least mitochondria are red blood cells which have virtually none, and cartilage and skin which may have a few dozen.

Monoclonal Antibodies: Lab-cloned proteins that mimic the immune system's ability to target specific disease cells or molecules.

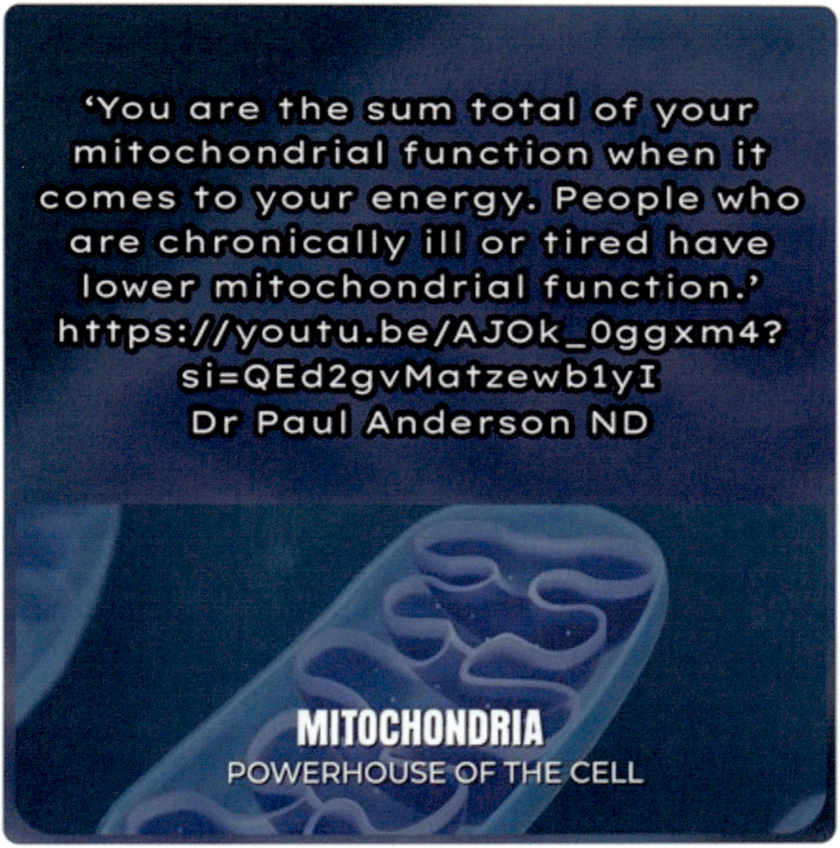

Morgellon's: The medical industry often denies this condition which involves synthetic filaments appearing from under the skin causing inflammation. According to Clifford Carnicon and industrial toxicologist Hildegarde Staninger, Morgellons comes from artificial spider-like webs which have been found draped over the countryside in some areas. It is not natural. When mainstream doctors don't understand what their patients are telling them, they have often been known to tell them that it's all in their heads.

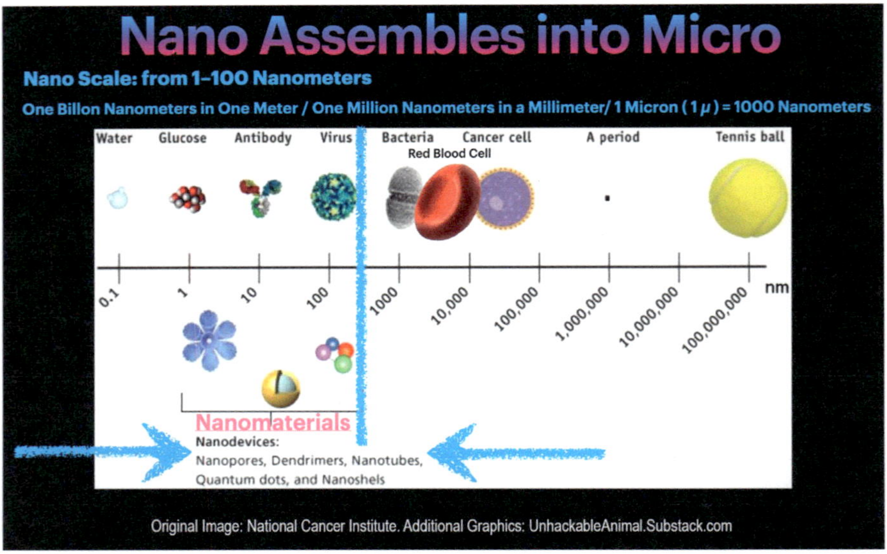

mRNA (messenger Ribo-Nucleic Acid): is a single-stranded molecule that carries genetic instructions from DNA to the cell's protein-making machinery (ribosomes) telling them how to make a specific protein.

*NAC. (N-Acetylcysteine): This boosts glutathione, the body's master antioxidant.

Nano: This is a measurement. One billionth of a metre, smaller than a cell but bigger than most atoms. They are so tiny they can go anywhere. We can't see things this size under most microscopes until they self-assemble into clusters and filaments.

Nano-dots: These appear in recent years as tiny blinking artificial lights in the blood of both vaccinated and vaccine-free people, some vaccines, dental anaesthetics, insulin and other substances. These appear to self-assemble into clusters and filaments in the blood

Nano-filaments: If the ones I saw in my blood were anything to go by, these assemble into what look like fluorescent ropes of fairy lights measuring about 5 microns in diameter. This new contamination is so small it can invade our bodies without our being aware of it. By the time we can see them in the blood, they have often assembled into structures larger than red blood cells.

Nanotechnology is a huge industry involving chemistry, biology, physics, engineering, medicine and electronics. Its aim is to program and control matter at the atomic scale.

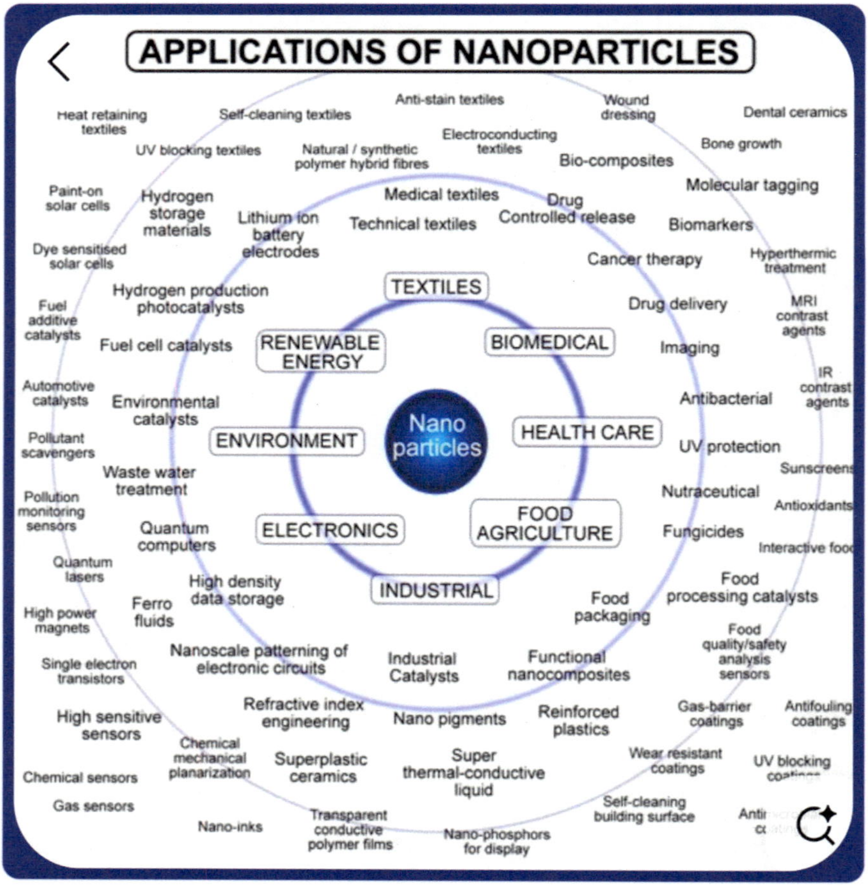

Naturopathy; a healing modality originally built solely on natural foundations. Naturopaths often try out treatments themselves before recommending them to patients. They take time to evaluate and listen to their patients and consider carefully how to heal with natural herbs, spices, quality supplements, diet, lifestyle and exercise.

*Neprinol: This is a supplement which includes nattokinase with serrapeptase and which may be useful in helping to keep fibrin and inflammation under control. Alkalinehealth.com.au

Nicotine: This is a substance found in tobacco. Our cells have nicotinic acetylcholine receptors which take up the snake venom toxins found in some of the covid shots. Using natural nicotine patches, gum or organic tobacco infusions in smoothies or even foot-baths has little risk, yet these may remove poisonous venoms and prevent new ones from entering the cells. This seems to improve brain and other issues.

Nootropic: A drug that improves the brain, memory and learning with low toxicity and few side effects.

Many people use this word to describe methylene blue.

ORF. Open Reading Frame: This is a part of a genetically engineered virus which is added to make it more harmful.

Orgonite: This is usually made from quartz crystal, copper or other metals and resin. It is sometimes made into beautiful pyramids and independent microscopists have found that it helps to disrupt EMF (Electro Magnetic Frequency) fields.

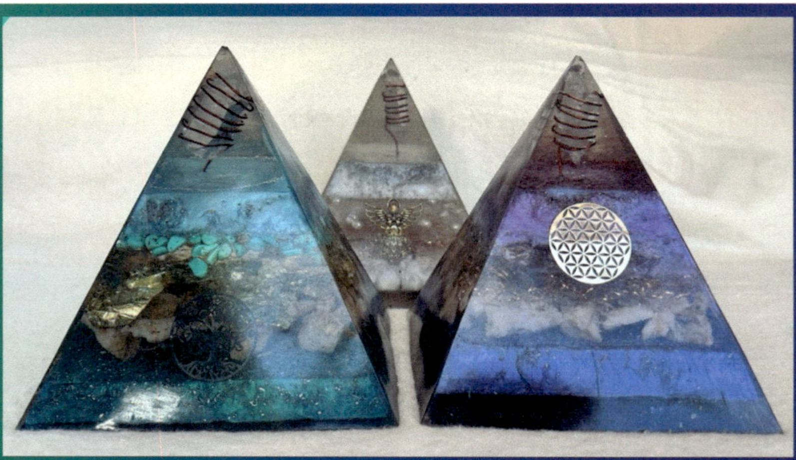

Orgonite pyramids help to disrupt EMF frequencies

Orthomolecular: a method of treatment that creates and maintains health with adequate levels of vitamins, minerals and amino acids. Over the years our soils and diets have often become lacking in the nutrients we need.

Ozone: Ozone is an inorganic molecule with three oxygen atoms. The extra oxygen atom is more available for the human body than the normal paired O2 oxygen molecules and looks for places in the body that need it. Ozone is not suitable to be inhaled in large quantities but can be used on the skin, in ozonated water or oils. It reduces inflammation and pathogens with a host of remedies. You can have ozone treatments at a clinic or invest in your own ozone generator.

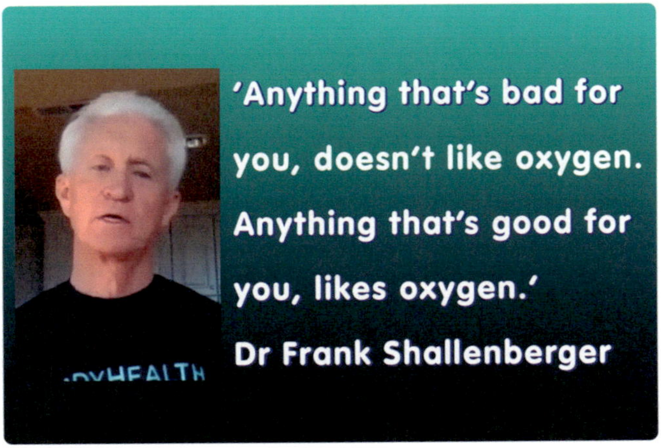

Parasites: Parasites can take many forms. They all poison us by secreting venoms and taking our nutrition and energy. It's becoming more and more accepted that many of us are carrying parasites within our bodies. In the post covid and chemtrail era, they are either natural or bio-engineered as stealth weapons. We usually think of them as being in the digestive tract, but they can also hide in blood, brain and organs. They steal nutrients from our bodies, excrete poisonous wastes and suck our energy.
They are harmful by definition.

*Paratrex: This is a powerful plant based anti-parasitic from Global Healing.

Pathogens: Any disease producing agents, such as bacteria or other micro-organisms.

Peptides: These are little chains of amino acids. They are regulators in the body and the building blocks of proteins.

Phase-contrast microscopy: This form of microscopy adds clarity to internal details of cells and other living samples.

Phosphorylation: This is adding phosphorous to a molecule or protein which can affect cell signals and regulation.

Photo-biomodulation: Any of several therapeutic techniques that use low-level laser light to relieve pain or to heal wounds.

*Pine needle essential oil: This is a natural disinfectant and that fresh, uplifting pine scent in your home actually gives some protection against mould, fungus and other pathogens.

Pyrazines: Some of the dozens of chemicals which are added to commercial cigarettes to make them addictive.

Plasma: 1: The pale fluid in which red and white blood cells and other elements in the blood are suspended.

Plasma: 2: Plasma is the fourth state of matter along with the other three: solid, liquid and gas. It's a gas in which electrons are separated from the nucleus of the atoms creating charged particles. These conduct electricity and respond to magnetic fields. Examples are lightning, the sun, neon lights and your tv screen.

Plasmids: Small DNA molecules that can replicate independently. They are used in genetic engineering to insert genes into cells.

Pleomorphism. This is the ability of yeasts to change into bacteria, or bacteria to change into yeasts in response to their environment. It was first spoken of by Antoine Bechamp in 1866 and observed by Royal Raymond Rife with his powerful microscopes in the 1920s and 1930s.

Polymer: A large molecule made up of repeating subunits called monomers. We might think of a polymer like a necklace, while the monomers are the individual beads. They can be natural like proteins or synthetic like plastics.

Polystyrene: (Styrofoam), The material our fragile mail-order deliveries might be packed in. Maria Crisler has actually identified this in some falls of what appeared at first glance to be snow.

Poly vinyl alcohol. (PVA) This is often a water-soluble white powder and is used in glues, packaging-films and pharmaceuticals.

*Potassium: This essential nutrient is found in many herbs and spices, sun dried tomatoes and beans. Some of the chemtrails contain the metal cesium which can displace essential potassium in the body.

Prions: These are badly folded proteins in the brain. Instead of being long and pliable like a chain they become contaminated and tangled up into knots so they don't perform as well. Parkinson's and Alzheimer's disease are associated with prions.

Psychic reader: In the same way that our dogs are much more sensitive to smell than we are, some people are much more sensitive to unseen worlds and messages around us. Depending on their particular talents, genuine psychic readers can help us connect with our higher selves and what we might call our guardian angels or our soul family in various ways.

Quantum dots. These are only 2-10 nanometers in size and assemble into fluorescent fairy-lights which can be seen blinking in the blood of humans, animals, and various injectables such as dental anaesthetics and insulin. According to Grok Ai They are used to label and track cells, proteins or drugs in the body. They weren't normally seen before 2022.

Redox: An abbreviation of reduction-oxidation where one molecule loses an electron and the other one gains it. Redox reactions occur in metabolism, photosynthesis and corrosion.

Reiki: A therapy from Japan which translated means 'spiritually guided life force energy.' It can treat the whole person spiritually, emotionally, physically and mentally, including past-life memories. The veil is thinning at this point in our history and (as I discovered myself) Reiki can be very powerful to clear traumatic and memorable past life incidents.

Rouleau: In terms of what goes on in the blood, rouleau is one of the stages where the blood cells start to lose their negative charge. They clump together and overlap in lines that look like little caterpillars. This prevents oxygen reaching the cells and can create conditions conducive to cancer.

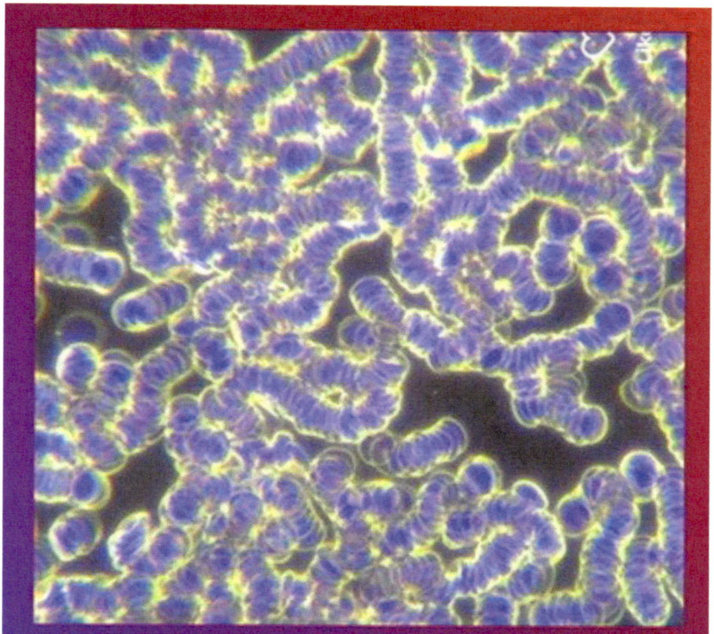

Rouleau formation in the blood

Sauna: The heat of a sauna allows the body to sweat out nano-toxins though the skin so they don't need to be excreted though the liver and kidneys.

Self-Assembly: The nano-filaments and hydrogels in our blood are often seen to assemble themselves, even after our death.

Silicon: Often found in chemtrail deposits, Silicon is a hard, shiny, grey material used as a conductor of electricity in computer chips.

Sodium Citrate: This is a salt of citric acid used as a food additive. In a medical setting it acts as an anti-coagulant in blood collection by binding calcium ions, preventing clotting.
It is used as a pharmaceutical antacid.

Solfeggio tones: These are coherent sounds often used in ancient musical traditions such as chanting. These are generally beneficial to the body.

Spherocytes: These are abnormalities of the blood which have become more common in the last couple of years. Normal red blood cells are fairly flat and concave in the middle, like a deflated rubber football. Spherocytes are slightly smaller and round like an inflated ball. This is usually due to toxins or anaemia.

Spike Protein: These words are controversial. Spike proteins are often illustrated as the surface of a virus which allow it to attach and enter cells. They are the 'keys' which allow viruses to unlock and enter human cells. Misfolded proteins seem to be an important part of this mystery.

*Supercharged C60: This is manufactured by Global Healing and helps to maintain optimal cell function and general vitality. Dr Ana Milhacea tells us that it protects against EMFs.

Tri-vortex technology: (Green Laser) This changes the structure of liquids from chaotic and disorganised to structured and flowing. Used properly, this benefits the body, in particular the red blood cells which become stronger and more capable of performing as they need.

Venoms: Scientific companies reproduce and manufacture large amounts of venoms based on snakes, snails, spiders and other poisonous creatures from around the world. They are said to be developed for therapeutic results but some researchers are suspicious of this claim. It appears that they have been used in some of the covid shot batches. Venoms like this can cause either clotting or thinning of the blood and various neurological issues.

Vesicle: A small sac containing fluid in the blood.

Viruses: These are controversial in today's world.

- Some doctors and researchers tell us that they don't exist.
- One definition tells us that viruses are nano sized infectious agents that can only multiply in the living cells of a host organism such as our body.
- We are told in documented detail by researcher Greg Harrison that enemies of humanity have been genetically modifying viruses to be increasingly deadly.

Draw your own conclusions.

Vitamin C: A wonderful healer which only human beings and guinea pigs are unable to produce in our own bodies. It can be used in large doses to bring oxygen to the cells, lower inflammation, heal wounds, help the body fight infections and overcome toxicity. Infections cause the body to use large amounts of vitamin C.

Weber Technology. (Green Laser). Used correctly this benefits the body by activating stem cells, releasing nitric oxide and telomerase and improving mood.

*Wild crafted wormwood (similar to Ivermectin) Protects the nicotine receptors from the venoms.

Zeolite: This is a blend of silicon and aluminium with a porous structure. It is often used in purification as it absorbs pollutants.
It may have been useful as a therapeutic for heavy metal detox before 2022 but many microscopists now report that it makes the nanotech in our bodies worse. Because of this I suggest that it should be used with great caution at this time.

Zeta potential: A measurement of the electrical charge on the outside of particles suspended in a liquid. Like a magnet, a positive charge attracts and a negative charge repels. Red blood cells need a negative zeta potential of about 30-50 millivolts to keep them bouncing off each other and flowing freely. If the zeta potential is too low – say near zero, or between -5 to +5 millivolts – it can lead to clumping and clotting.

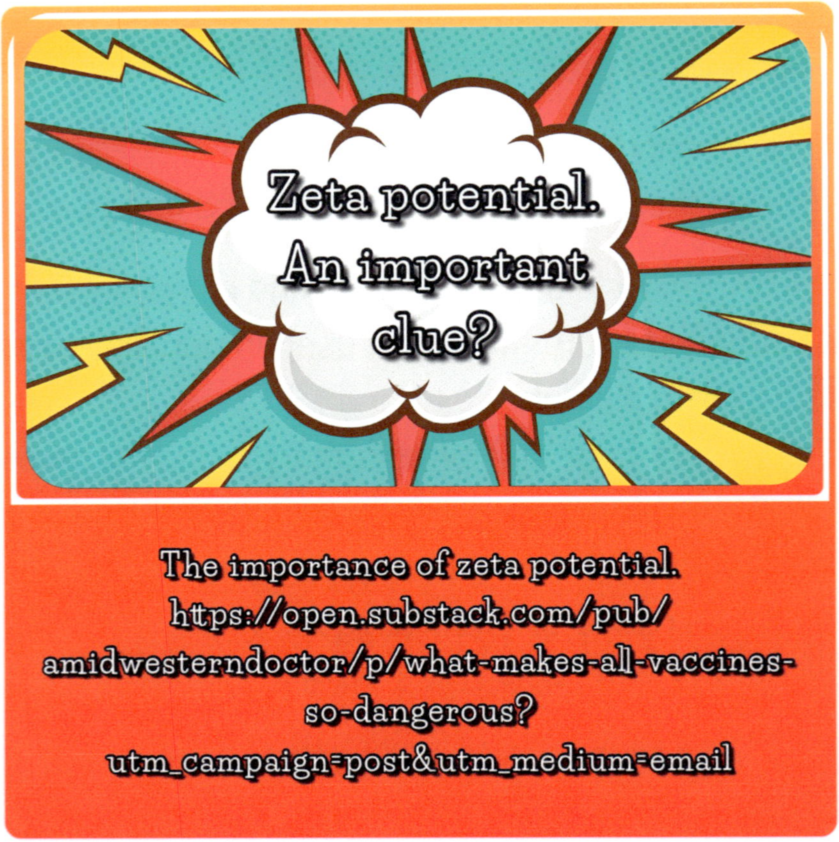

*Zinc: This is considered an essential nutrient as the body can't make it on its own. It has many functions in the body including skin issues, blood sugar and insulin regulation.

The :lood

It all starts with my own story.

I have a motor home and took a trip up the East coast of Australia in 2024 to talk about my books, the 4th edition of 'Vaccines, Myths and Facts' and 'Detox after Covid and Thrive' to various groups and gatherings all the way up to the Sunshine Coast. It was great connecting with old and new friends along the way and I was hanging out at my favourite old haunts in Queensland when I happened to see a local naturopath who ran Oligoscan spectroscopy blood testing.

With the Oligoscan, the practitioner puts the sensor on your non-dominant hand and you get an instant simple read out of your metal toxicity, vitamin and mineral levels. I first came across it at a health retreat in the US over ten years ago and I've loved the idea and immediate simplicity of this non-invasive blood test ever since.

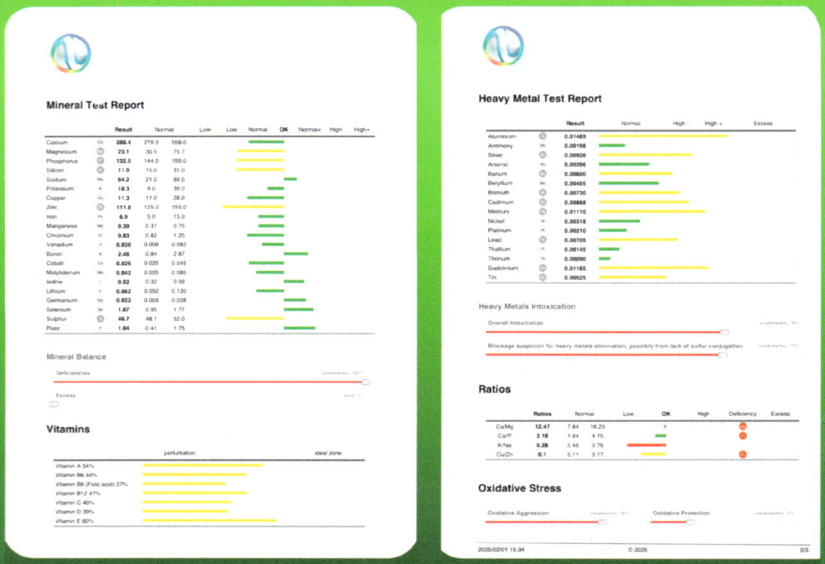

The Oligoscan: instant, non invasive check for minerals and heavy metals in the blood.

The naturopath did the test and confidently went through the supplements I was taking, recommending high quality all-natural organic brands. I was vaccine free, I hadn't taken any other medication for a couple of decades, and all was good.

I noticed that she also offered live blood analysis, sometimes known as dark field microscopy. This is another fascinating and relatively rare test which (when done properly and with care) shows in real time the health of the living cells of your blood. It's a swirling world of insight from a single, carefully collected pinprick.

This is another test I have believed in since I heard Tony Robbins talking about it on his Living Health program twenty years ago. I bought his CD audio set and listened to it in the car dozens of times. I can still hear his big husky voice communicating powerfully to us that that the health of our bodies is dependent on the health of our cells.

It always made sense to me, I'd had live blood analysis done a few times back then and my blood had always been pretty much picture-perfect with free flowing, well formed, nice round cells. This was my own base-line memory for how healthy blood should look. The naturopath had been doing these tests for several years and I jumped at the chance to check my blood again, expecting to see this …

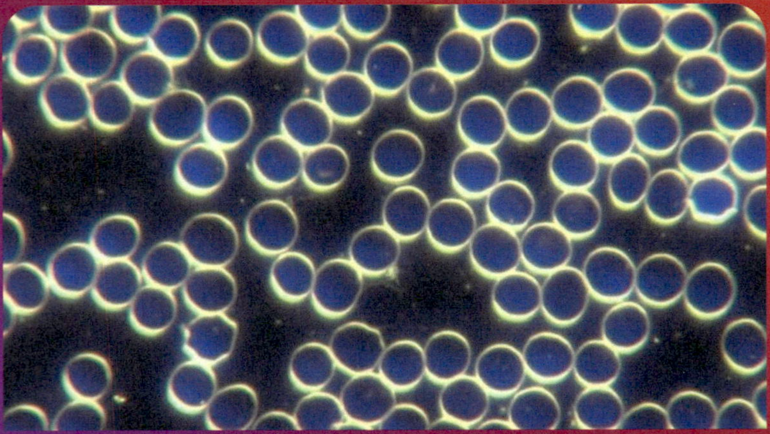

Normal live blood.

Except that this time my blood wasn't flowing freely

In spite of my relatively healthy diet and lifestyle, my blood was sticking together in chain-like rouleau formations. It wasn't moving around as it should and I was horrified to see quite large fluorescent tube-like filaments on the screen which were causing even more clumping. Some of my white blood cells were clinging limply to these things in a sad attempt to get rid of them, obviously without success.

It's pretty clear that our blood isn't supposed to have fluorescent ropes of fairy lights or mysterious dark pools of hydrogel in it.

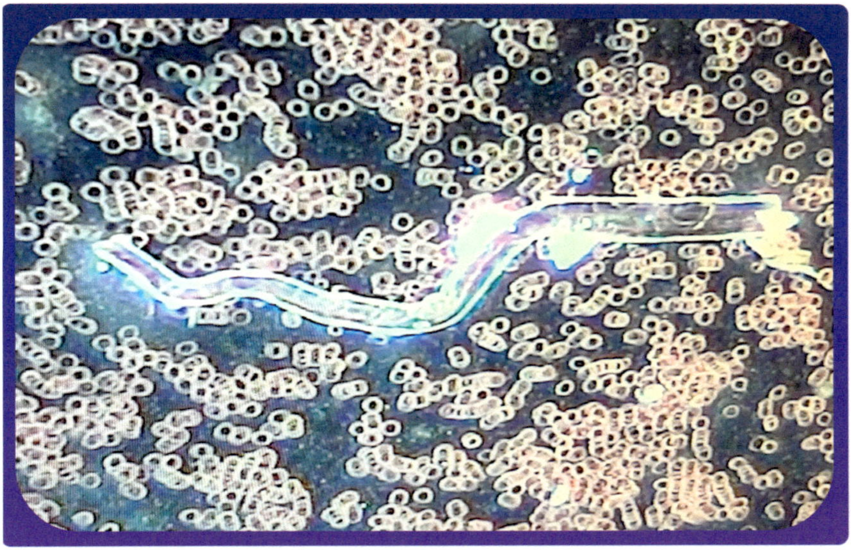

I was shocked. I looked from the screen to my previously confident, brisk and super fit naturopath. She wilted a bit.

'My blood's the same,' she almost whispered.
'So is my husband's. I'm afraid to check the kids.
Most people are like this now.

I don't know how to get rid of them.'

We stared at each other.

A whiff of hopelessness wafted into the room and drifted mockingly around our years of education, proactive health regimes, carefully crafted supplements and positive outlooks.

I didn't want to etch this clumpy image into my brain in case I somehow manifested more of it. I refused screenshots, not thinking in the moment that I was going to write a book about it all. I had seen all I wanted to see.

Looking back, I'm so grateful to this experienced and accomplished naturopath for her complete openness and honesty. She could have shown me other parts of the slide, or told me it was something more commonplace and nothing to worry about, but she didn't. She told me the truth.

Her reaction alone that day told me clearly that this was new, different, unwanted and potentially here to stay.

I was in shock for a few days while the enormity of this discovery sank in … Were these fluorescent things going to lead to blood clots? Would they find their way to my heart? How could they possibly squeeze through the tiny capillaries of my eyes, lungs and fingertips where the blood flows one cell at a time? Were they going to get worse? Were they going to grow into the rubbery clots I'd seen London undertaker and embalmer John O'Looney talking about? Was I going to have a stroke? Was I going to have a heart attack? Was I going to die?

Then there was the bigger picture: Where were they coming from? Not only had I not been vaccinated but I had deliberately had little close contact with anyone who had. Did everyone have them? If they were in the air, were they in the water, on the fields and in those carefully tended rows of organic vegetables I loved to buy at the farmers' markets?

As I learned later … They were everywhere.

Microchipped?

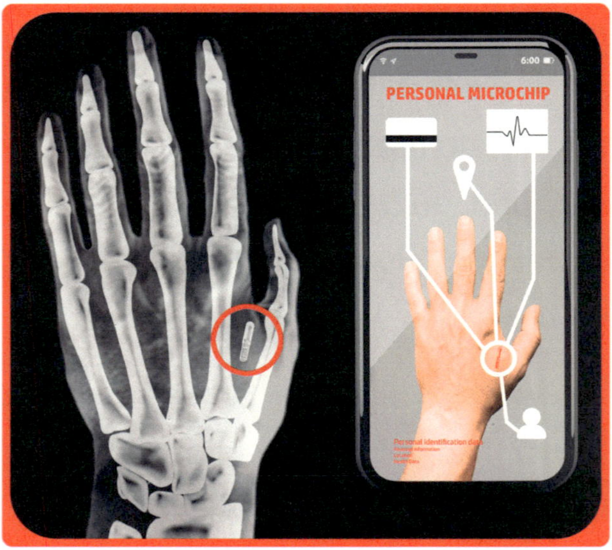

Whatever happened to those conversations we had a few years ago when we all decided we didn't want to be micro-chipped like dogs? It seems that once again, we've been completely ignored by government agencies. Manufacturers have designed technologies so infinitesimally tiny that we could breathe them in or absorb them through our eyes, pores and tissues without us even knowing. We don't need anyone to insert a big micro-chip under our skin if the antennae are nano-sized and already assembling and growing in our bodies.

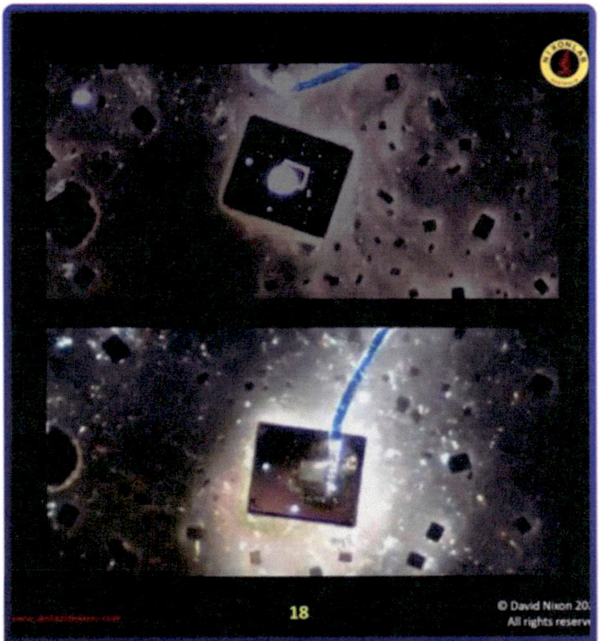

A closer look at the same Pfizer Comirnaty shot. Two photos, (200 x magnification) taken by Dr David Nixon, two days apart: 7th (top) and 9th December 2022.
Journal of Bionanotechnocracy
Volume 1, Issue 1 - April 2025.
Active Microscale Construction in Pfizer Comirnaty: Investigating Complex Self-Assembling Structures.
https://drdavidnixon.com/1/en/topic/volume-1-issue-1-april-2025

It took a few days for all this to sink in and for me to register that in fact I still seemed to have as much energy as ever and wasn't suffering any apparent ill effects in everyday life. I walked on the glorious beaches of the Sunshine Coast and still felt great. I am eternally grateful for this, and I soon pulled myself around to my usual positive mindset.

That didn't alter the fact that those shiny ribbon things still didn't belong there. They didn't belong in my blood and they don't belong in yours.

I believe that over 90% of the Australian population, vaccinated and vaccine free alike, including children, have these filaments in their blood without even knowing it. I believe the situation is the same in North America, Canada, the UK and, possibly to a lesser extent, Europe.

This is confirmed by statements made by some of the dedicated teams working to clear them. Many people in the field claim that everyone is now contaminated.

I had seen these shiny nano-filaments before.

Dr Ana Milhacea has a clinic which physically removes or controls these contaminants with intravenous EDTA (more on this later). She is active on her Substack page where she talks about her photographs of these filaments and other formations, collected from around the world. I had seen these when I wrote Detox after Covid and Thrive, but I hadn't really taken them too seriously before, especially as, at the time, she seemed to offer no simple solutions.

When I found that my own blood looked exactly like the backdrop to her podcasts, I really began to pay attention.

She talked about being able to clear them physically but she is in the US and her clinical methods for clearing the blood with intravenous EDTA chelation therapies are highly specialised, inevitably expensive, and on the other side of the world.

I was still pondering all this when I visited Eumundi Markets a couple of days later. My friends Alyce and Larry have a stall there selling a variety of high-quality remedies they make themselves in their factory under the name of Miracle Products. I had used their nascent iodine for years and I knew them both to be extremely well researched and knowledgeable about their products. Still shaken by what I had seen in my blood, I told my story.

Alyce listened carefully and immediately said: 'Methylene-blue. One drop for every four kilos of body weight per day, in filtered water.'

It sounded like a plan …

I already had some of their high-quality BluZone, 1% methylene blue with me and had been taking a small number of drops most days. 'That won't do anything,' she said confidently. 'You need enough to do the metabolic repair. For your weight you need thirteen drops a day.'

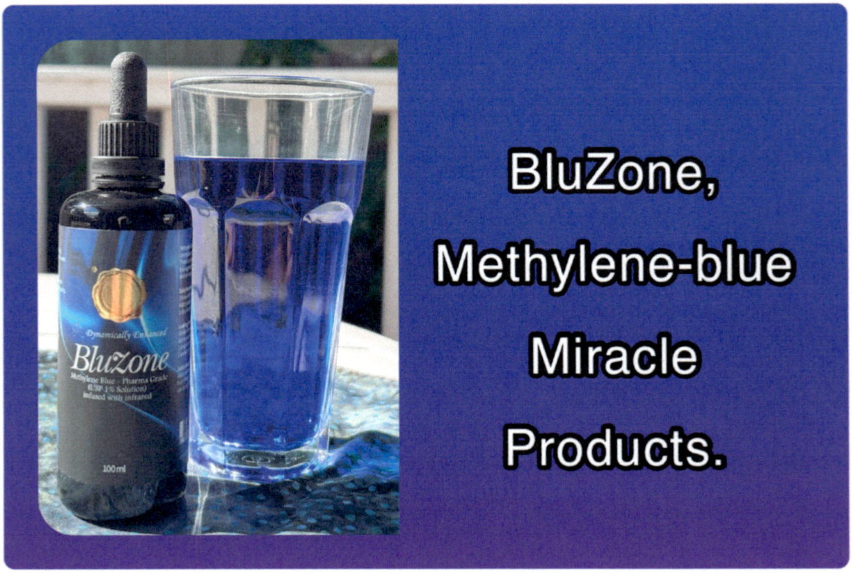

In the absence of any alternatives, and on the road in my motor home, that's exactly what I did.

I was already taking an array of quality supplements including those supplied by my first practitioner.

These supplements might have helped clear the fluorescent nano-filaments, but I believe in my case that the majority of the effect in the first six months was due to Methylene Blue.

I have so many favourite beaches, haunts and friends along the East Coast of Australia that I took my time heading South towards home and stayed for a while in Newcastle, catching up with people and watching the cargo ships sail in and out of the harbour.

My good friend recommended a local naturopath and live blood analysis practitioner and I met Kirsty Bednar from EmpowerU Natural Health for the first time.

After around six weeks of religiously taking BluZone methylene blue and the other supplements I was keen to know how the shiny nano-filaments were going. Kirsty had been doing live blood analysis for over a decade and was very thorough, carefully counting the numbers of red blood cells, white blood cells, fat molecules, parasites, inflammation and other elements, I had some parasite activity and the nano filaments were still there, but approximately 30% less.

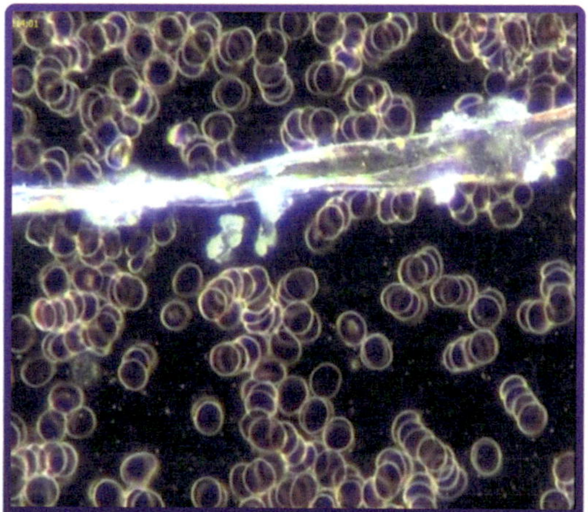

My blood:
Microscopy by Kirsty Bednar:
11 October 2024.
A typical early shot with white blood cells clinging to the nano-filaments. I had been taking daily methylene-blue and there were a lot less nano-filaments like this to be seen in the blood at this stage.

This was encouraging news indeed.
This looked like the start of the next book.
A book that people didn't know they needed yet.

How could they unless they too were able to look into the microscopic world of their own cells?

At this stage, a few of you may not believe that nano-filaments and strange clusters of fairy ropes in the blood are even real.

I wish you were right. More on this later ....

A family holiday and Christmas came and went. In mid-January 2025, after taking BluZone and other supplements religiously every single day, I suddenly muscle tested that I should take a break from it. I now believe that I might have been overloading my liver not with the BluZone itself, but with what was being cleared from the blood. The suggestions I share with you later in the book pay more attention to the wellbeing of the liver and microbiome.

I decided to make the trip back to Newcastle to see Kirsty Bednar again in February 2025. Live blood analysis is such a finely tuned glimpse into our inner workings and specialists are a rare breed. I'm so glad I decided to return to the same practitioner and compare like with like. After another three months, the filaments were still shiny, but only about 10-15% of them remained. My blood was flowing well, and – as a huge side benefit - the parasite activity had disappeared.

Great News!

Now it was definitely time to write a book the world didn't know it needed.

I decided to continue with the BluZone for a while as a living experiment. and start writing about this and other possible detox options of the post covid and chemtrail era.

At this stage I had a reading with my trusted psychic and dear friend. She has connected with my guides to steer me deftly through many challenges and triumphs over ten years. She suggested that I should do methylene blue 8 days on and 8 days off. (I'll expand on this later in the book and offer some initial recommendations for you.)

Natural Healing

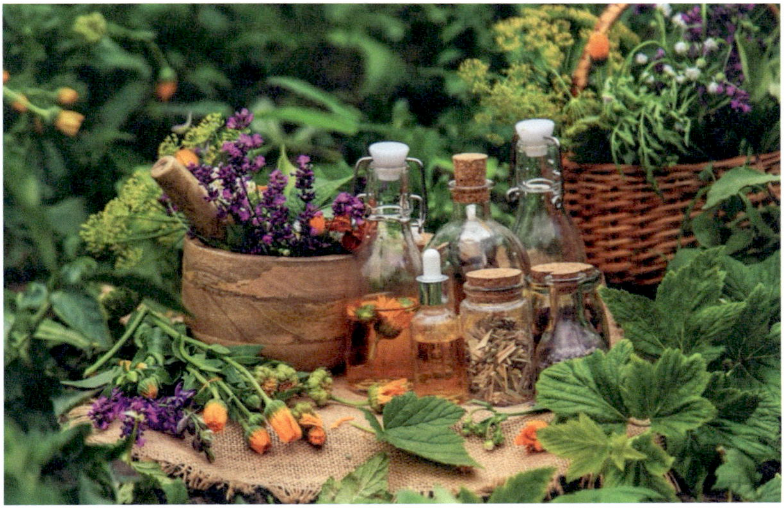

Mankind has a rich heritage of tried and trusted natural health remedies and practices that have served our cultures for generations. Among them are herbs, spices, teas, oils, tinctures, supplements, breath, prayer, meditation, sound healing, clean water, exercise, gratitude and immersing ourselves in nature in a variety of ways. It's the solid foundation of herbalism, naturopathy and traditional remedies from around the world. Strengthening ourselves wisely with these traditional health-giving practices is and will always be the foundation of health. The stronger and more resilient we are in body, mind and spirit, the better we will fare, even in these uncertain times.

Another naturopath friend expands on this. 'When someone comes to see me for the first time, I like to do a full bloodwork check and other tests to gather as many clues as possible to check the whole system for underlying deficiencies and imbalances.

Some people may have suffered more during health challenges, including covid shots, because the foundation of their health wasn't as strong as it might have been. They may have tried to use supplements on an ad hoc basis to support their bodies, but haven't been aware of the whole picture. The human body is very complex and finely balanced. Everything affects everything else, especially as we age.'

I realised this for myself on this journey, as Kirsty wisely encouraged me to do a full blood test and overall check. Like so many of us, I've lost trust in mainstream doctors and have steered clear of their offices for many years, but, being in apparent good health, hadn't seen a naturopath for a full check either.

I'm glad I did. It was the most thorough health check I'd ever had. We all know we have to service our vehicles to catch potential issues before they cause problems and I think the same principle applies to our bodies. It's an interesting journey, and I'm very grateful for this detour and wake-up call. I'm now eating (even) better and I'm back at the gym working away to maintain those all-important muscles.

'The beautiful thing about your body is that it always wants to get better. We're the ones suppressing it by feeding it junk, exposing it to toxins, and not allowing it to do what it's designed to do.
Every disease starts with toxicity in the internal and external environment. But if you give the body what it needs and remove what it doesn't, it will naturally return to balance.
It's built to regenerate.
Your body knows exactly what to do.'
Dr Ed Group, Chiropractor, Naturopath

However, I believe that the trusted basics may no longer be enough. They are wonderful as a foundation but the world has changed. We are entering a new paradigm with new attacks on our health.

A phrase from the Wizard of Oz springs to mind...

Somewhere near the start of their journey Dorothy says to her little dog Toto …

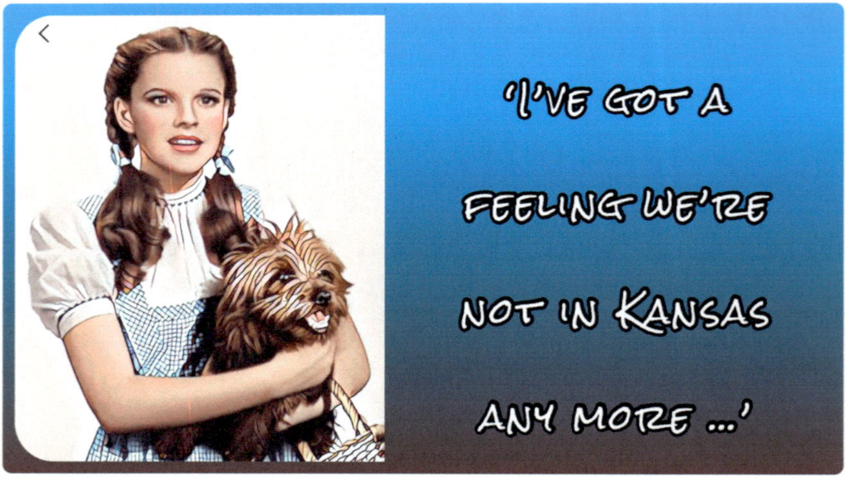

New spanners have been thrown in the works and the fact is that we don't know what the future holds for us all.

I have focussed on the nano-micro filaments as my entry into this strange world, but there are other new threats for us to consider in this era: Chemtrail cocktails, genetically modified pathogens, snake venoms, and turbo cancers

'The presence of these new assaults means that we may all need to open our minds and study this contamination and its remedies in a new light. There have to be more remedies to all this. We just have to take our blinkers off and find them.

Maybe we are being invited to look outside our old paradigms?

Maybe we are being invited to view this precious life from a new perspective?

Maybe we are being invited to study the live, moving cells of our blood more closely?

Maybe we are being invited to open our minds and collaborate with other researchers?

Maybe we are being challenged to bear witness to it all, even when it means the end of lucrative careers?

> *Maybe we are being invited to research light and sound frequency more closely as healing tools?*
>
> *Maybe we are being invited to use our intention to influence more of what is happening in our bodies?*
>
> *Maybe we are being invited to become more acquainted with our intuition, our higher selves and our God?*
>
> *Maybe we are being invited to purify ourselves physically, mentally, emotionally and spiritually in order to usher in a new Earth?*
>
> *Maybe we are being challenged to be brave?*
>
> *Maybe we are being pushed to the cliff edge so we can fly?*

In this book, along with the wise words of researchers and strange microscopic images, I'll be combining information from my own muscle testing, from a kinesiologist, and a psychic reader. I've been using insights like this to help me navigate my way through life for over ten years. I believe it's time these talents and skills were brought into more mainstream awareness, especially as the skilled practitioners we really need to tackle this onslaught on our health are still as rare as hens' teeth. For the most part, we're on our own.

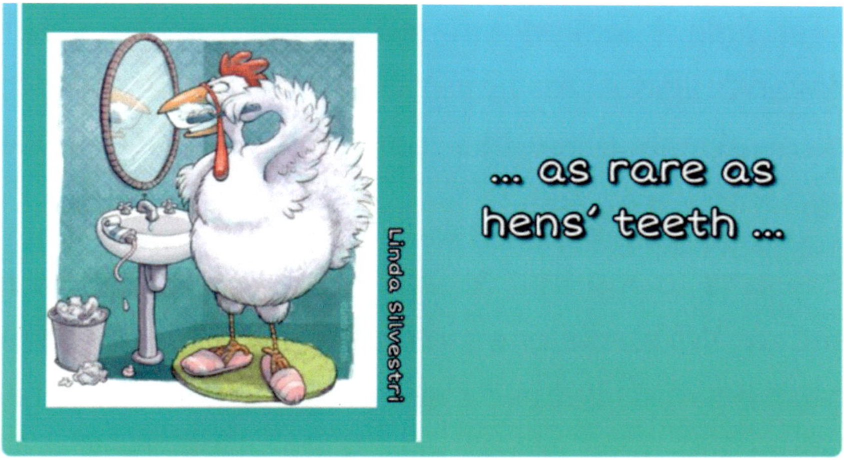

I also very cautiously asked a few basic questions of Ai.

Ai

I dipped my toe in the Ai water for the first time for some of the definitions. This is an interesting journey in itself. It can be spectacularly right, but it was also spectacularly wrong several times on basic facts which magnified my suspicion of it enormously. A friend told me it could have written the whole book in ten minutes. I'm sure it could, but that would be cheating and I wouldn't trust it as far as I could throw it…

Last time I looked I'm still a real person and I haven't used Ai for any of the writing, preferring to painstakingly piece this journey together sentence by sentence myself.

It seems to me that Ai isn't much different from a satnav, Wikipedia or even a calculator. These are all good servants but bad masters. They are amazingly useful but most of us have learned the hard way that we have to be aware of the overview before we follow their guidance.

Before we trust that maths calculation, we have to use our own brains to know if we are looking at an answer of around 200 or 2,000. Before we plug an address into our satellite navigation gizmo, we need to cross check the approximate route we are following so we don't find ourselves heading north when we really wanted to drive south. Most of us know that Wikipedia is useful for some basic facts, but dreadful for intelligent assessment of any given situation. I think if we can use Ai with the same discernment, to *help* us rather than *replace* us, we should be ok.

Some of us may remember the classic film '2001, A Space Odyssey'. Hal, the computer, runs the space ship perfectly until Dave, the astronaut, is outside the ship doing routine maintenance and Hal decides he doesn't need him any more. He locks him out and the last time we see poor old Dave, he's floating off into space never to be seen again …

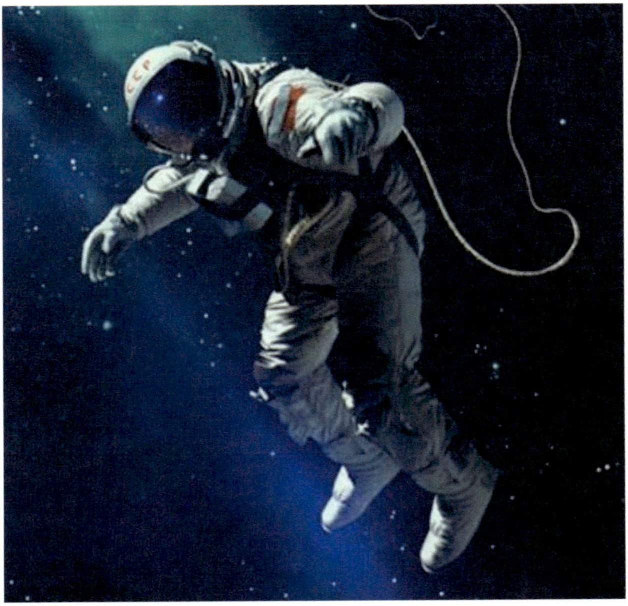

Since I first wrote this a few short weeks ago, as predicted, the Ai I was using had indeed run amok. Far from the reliable, balanced and honest research assistant it seemed to be at first, I had to be careful because of its occasional tendency to ignore facts in favour of tired old propaganda.

That was quick. Glad I didn't trust it with my space ship.

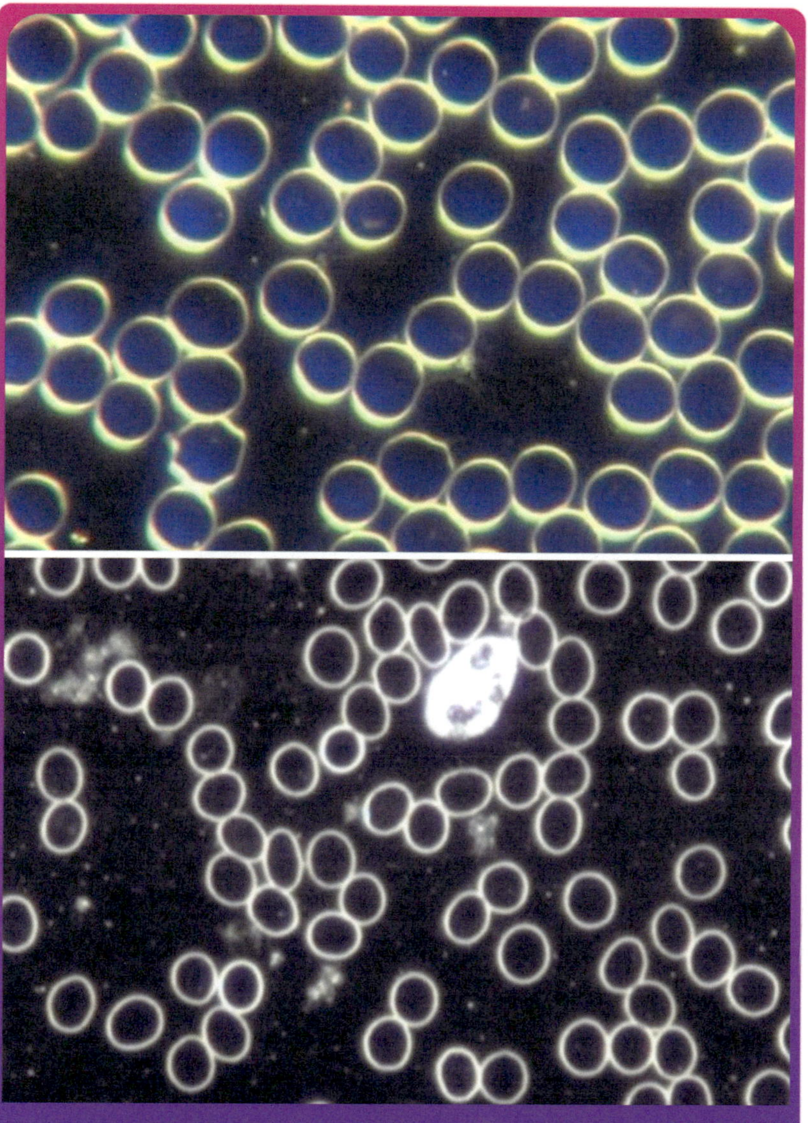

Normal blood.
Nice, round, free-flowing cells

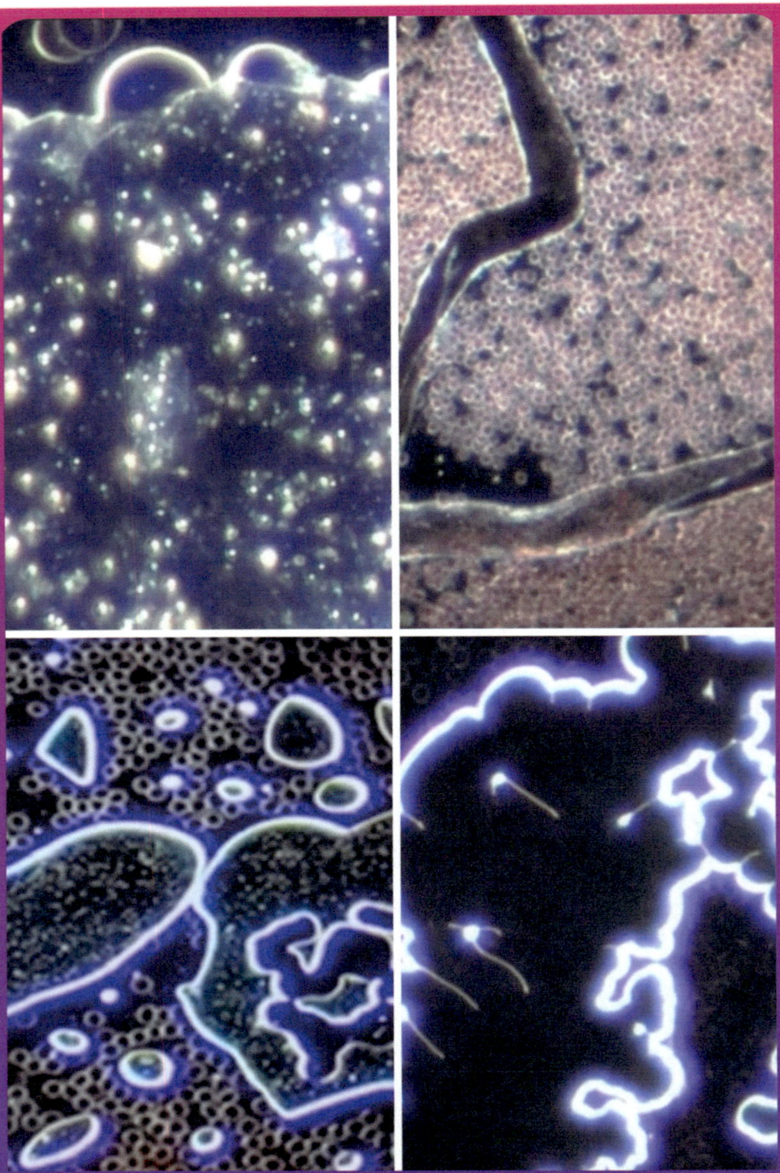

Blood contamination.
Photography: Dr Sandy Corlett.

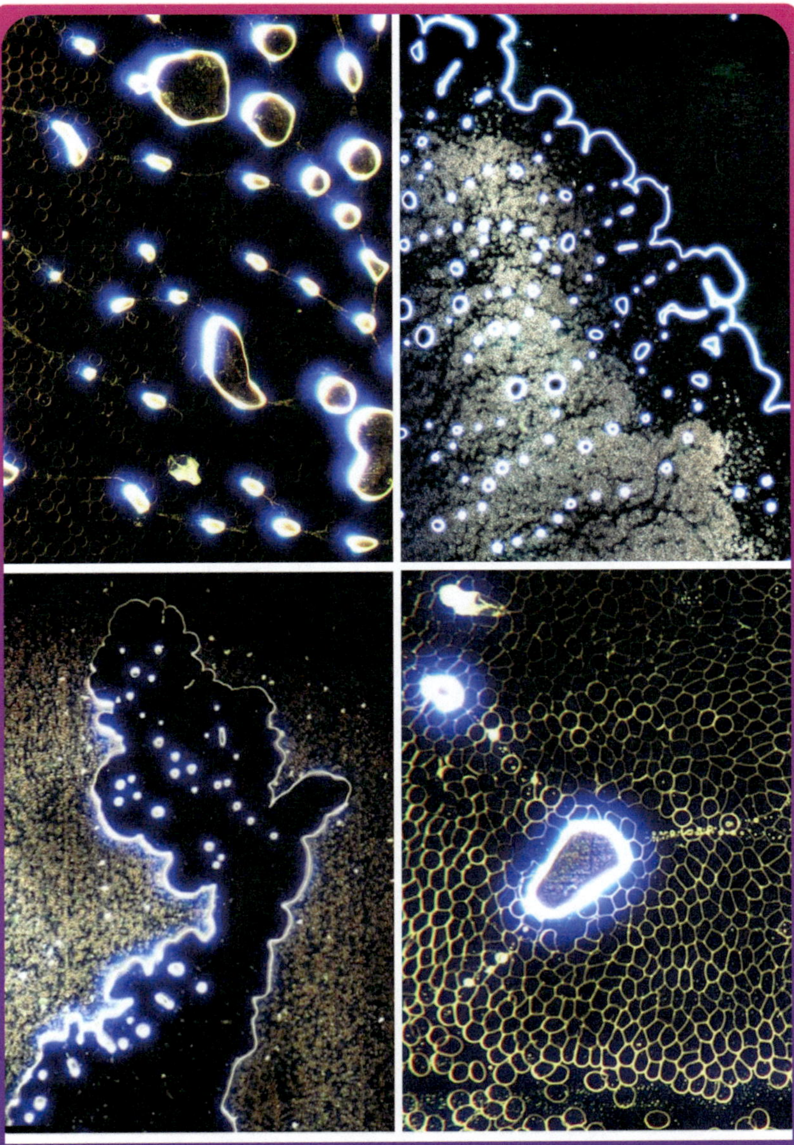

Blood contamination.
Photography. Dr David B Nixon.

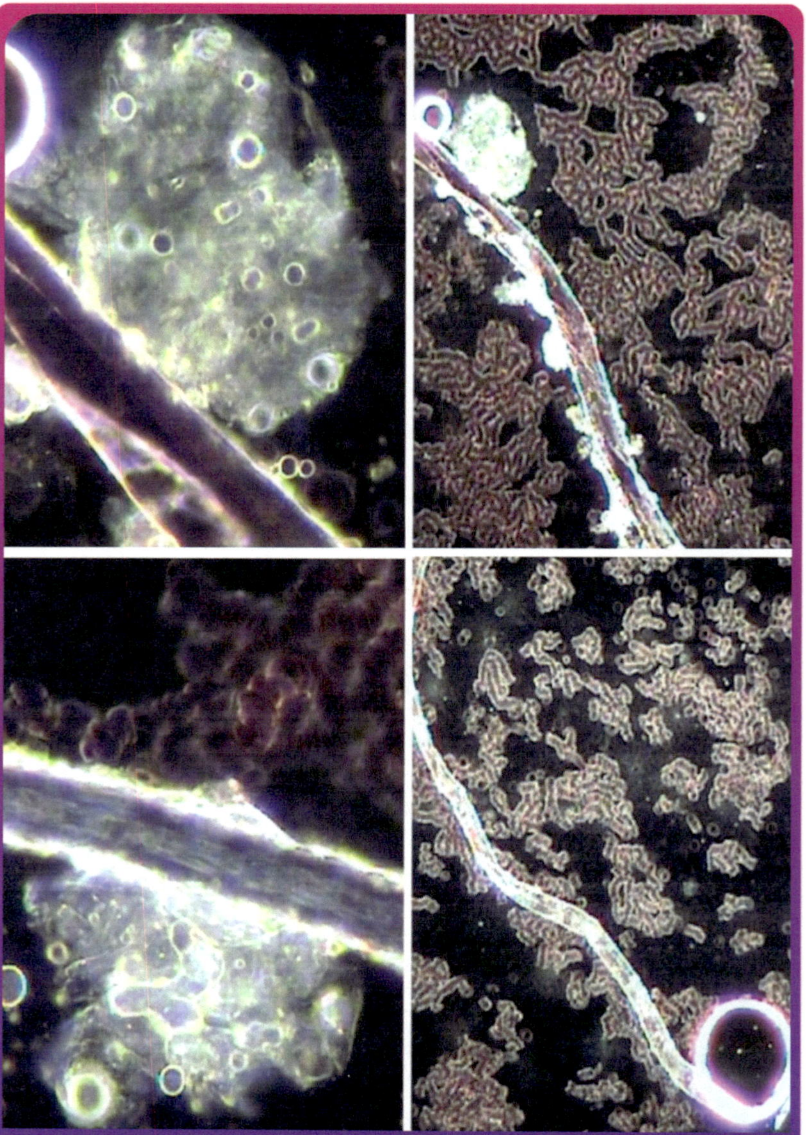

My blood contamination
Photography: Kirsty Bednar ND, BHSc (Comp Med)

Nano-filaments

A tiny handful of people had spotted this blood contamination occasionally before 2020, Clifford Carnicom, Elena Freeland, Hildegarde Staninger, Harvey Bigelsen and Tony Pantalleresco spring to mind. However, it was very rare, and none of the professionals I know had seen it before 2021. Some Naturopaths and professionals are finding that other remedies that were working well in 2022-23 aren't working quite as well now. Their patients are still struggling and it's often hard to work out why. There are other tried and tested remedies (like zeolite) which used to be considered safe, but which appear to react badly with this new contamination.

To complicate matters even further, many people don't even admit that these filaments are real, or new. There is a school of thought that they are holograms. If this were the case my poor, overwhelmed white blood cells wouldn't have been clinging to them as they were. There are live blood analysts who would like to believe they are due to a leaky gut. Anyone who has spent more than fifteen minutes listening to microbiologist Dr Ana Milhacea, Dr Sandy Corlett, Dr David Nixon, embalmer Richard Hirschman and many others, agree that this is not the case.

There are also people who will tell you that this vast array of new anomalies is due to imperfections in low quality slides or even lint on dirty slides. Trusted groups of dedicated micronauts around the world don't fall for that. Many of them have been looking at live blood, urine, vaccines, rainwater, and medications such as dental anaesthetics for decades. They invest in good quality slides, clean them carefully and take note of any imperfections before they start work. They know the difference between faulty slides and strange new contamination. Once the blood is on the slide, dedicated microscopists often photograph movement and development of structures and hydrogels over hours and days. They can see these shapes forming and changing before their eyes.

Dr David Nixon, now well known internationally as an experienced dark field microscopist has written a great paper on the reality of this new contamination: The Psyop that Wasn't. A Response, which you can find on the Nixonlab Substack.

The real clincher is to feel your very own rubbery clot, spun from a small vial of your very own blood. More on that later.

> 'Nanotechnology is not a fantasy.
> It is not a meme, a narrative, a virus, or a distraction.
> It is a well-documented, deeply invested field with extensive military, industrial and biomedical applications - and it now stands confirmed by direct observational evidence across multiple product categories and biological contexts.'
> Dr David Nixon, M.B., Ch.B.

I believe this nano technology in our blood is partially artificial. It appears to be intelligent and often continues to morph and grow long after normal blood on the slides has dried up and died.

I believe we all need to do something on a regular basis to prevent re-contamination and get it out of our bodies.

I think it's a good idea to think about it in the same way we might start going to the gym, taking more walks, going to the dentist, cleaning up our diet or visiting the chiropractor. I have a variety of options for you to work with later on in the book.

'Why would they do this to us ...?'

If you still find it hard to believe that our own governments, would use our own tax dollars to harm us, I do empathise.

It's a horrible thing to have to admit.

I remember a conversation with a friend several years ago when I had already written my first edition of 'Vaccines, Myths and Facts'. Speaking of vaccine damage in a hushed voice she asked, 'Is it deliberate?' It was something I had never really wanted to admit to myself before. There was no denying it. I replied in equally hushed tones, 'Yes.'

It's interesting how these big, ugly truths are often whispered, as if they are too awful to speak out loud.

Once I acknowledged this huge fact: That our governments are capable of committing crimes against humanity on an industrial scale and lying about it, I began to see other things more clearly. Once the trust is broken, we can't unsee it. We who had crossed this line long ago and abandoned trust in the system before covid was launched could see that it was a plandemic from the very start, even though we didn't understand exactly what form it would take.

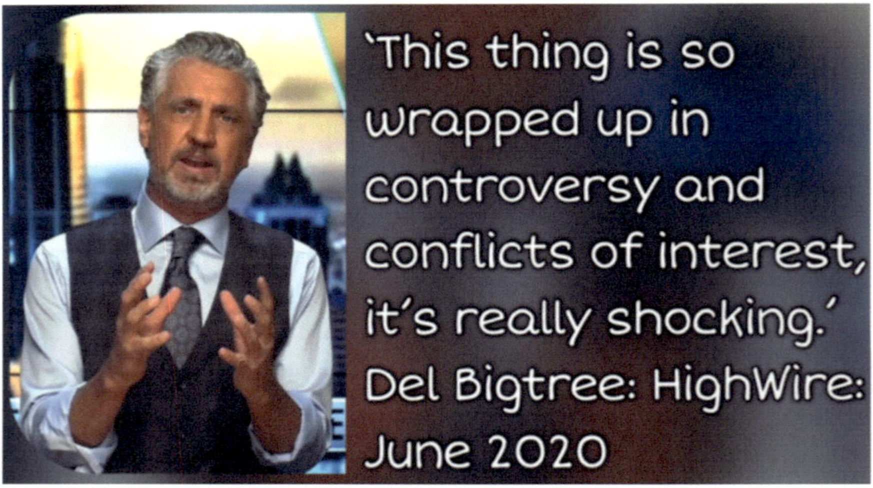

I have tracked the Australian death rates each year since 2015. In the four years following the jab roll out: 2022 to 2025 we have had over 107,000 excess deaths. That's more than the number of Australians killed in wartime.

An administrator at a large Australian city hospital confided to me recently that since the covid shots, their birth admissions are down to half the pre-covid numbers and yet the NICU (neonatal intensive care unit), for babies who are premature or struggling in some way, is busier than ever.

The hospital is overflowing and experienced Australian doctors and nurses are leaving the system rather than speaking out. They are being replaced with much younger and less experienced staff from overseas. These youngsters, fresh out of training and keen to make their way in a new country with a new career in a new language, are far less likely to speak out about what they see. They are far more likely to believe the narrative, do what they are told and go with the flow.

In the post-covid era, the evidence of harm is so overwhelming that there are millions of us who know. There is no going back.

Welcome to Stepford

Most of us are aware of the film 'The Stepford Wives.' For those that have missed the huge number of versions and releases of this film, the plot is very simple. A normal American family moves into a pleasant little town. They settle in and the wife soon notices that, although beautifully groomed and friendly, most of the women in the town are superficial, blank and strangely empty. She makes friends with one of the rare lively ones and is horrified when this woman is also suddenly transformed, losing her vibrant personality and sense of humour. It turns out that their husbands at the local men's association are secretly having their wives micro-chipped and turning them into compliant living robots. The films have various endings and I won't spoil them for you.

After learning about these issues for years, there's no escaping the conclusion that this seems to be pretty much what our governments (and those who control them) had planned for us for a long time …

: linkered Science?

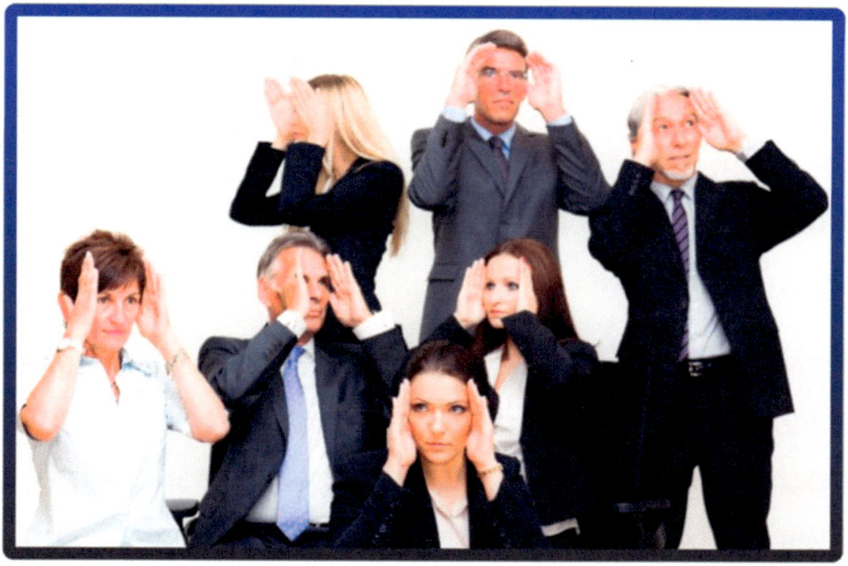

It's interesting to realise that a lot of science has been trimmed and packaged into controlled, predictable spaces by unseen powers over many decades and that this is now seriously impacting our ability to recover from or even recognise any new threats.

Firstly, scientists are usually trained to ignore and even ridicule the multi-dimensional nature of the universe, our innate powers of intuition, remote vision, psychic ability, and healing of physical wounds with the help of meditation, frequency and the presence of a creator God. We now know that even animals, plants and trees are able to sense many things beyond our limited comprehension.

As humankind, I believe we are magical beings made in the image of God. We are capable of many things that many of us have not yet allowed ourselves to even imagine.

Every aspect of formal university education steers us into specialised study. As academics, scientists and doctors rise up the ranks in their chosen, careers, their field of knowledge tends to become increasingly narrow. They begin to know more and more about less and less. They believe the papers peer-reviewed by biased industry insiders. They think they know all about the spine but may know nothing about the parasites that might be messing up the spinal fluid. They believe they know all about eyes but may know nothing about iridology or the effect of vaccine damage creating mini-strokes and preventing young eyes from tracking together. Sometimes, it seems, they can't even be bothered to look.

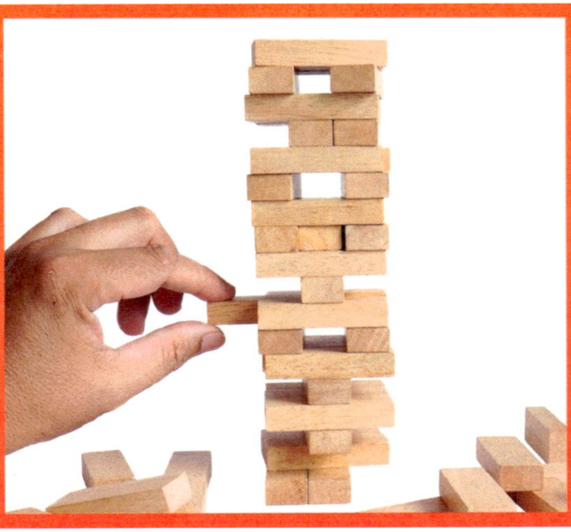

Ideas can be dangerous to established careers. A simple new solution to a complex old problem might topple a whole industry.

Many of the most insightful scientists work as independently of the system as they can and have often studied for two or more degrees in different fields. They often report that many issues are viewed very differently from one specialisation to another.

University Funding

University research is big business and funding is everything.

Most doctors and researchers are simply not looking for pioneering leading edge research that truly serves humanity. That might be risky.

There might not be any money in it. Simple answers might jeopardise their career. They're looking for projects that are safe and handsomely funded by the industries that benefit. These are the studies that lead to higher salaries, fame, fortune and even multi-million dollar patents and licensing agreements. This means that fundamental research challenging the status quo or seeking simple low-cost answers is often routinely ignored. In the words of Charlotte Gerson, daughter of natural cancer treatment pioneer Max Gerson talking about hydrogen peroxide:

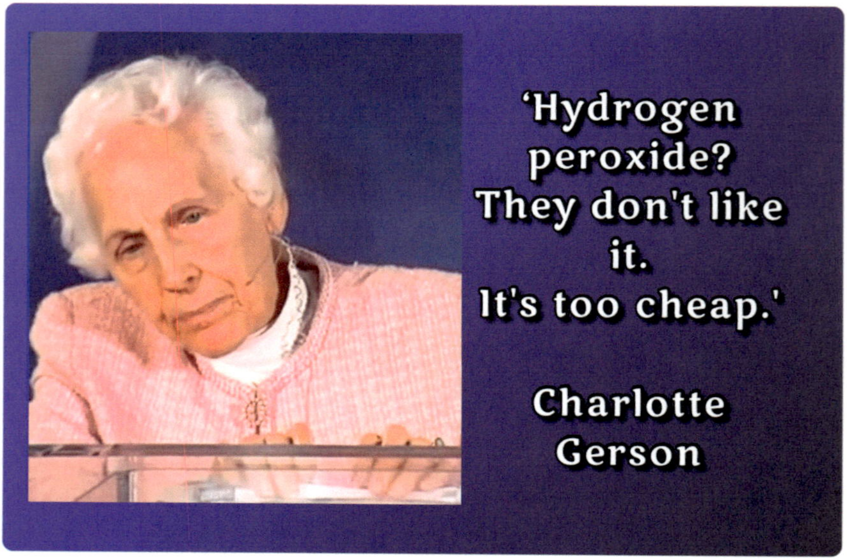

If doctors or researchers venture too deep into areas the pharmaceutical industry might want to keep secret, it can be ruinous for their careers. Professor Chris Exley (known world-wide as Mr Aluminium) was stripped of his title and life-long tenure at Keele university when he continued to pursue the connection between aluminium and brain damage in Alzheimer's and autism. Pediatrician, Dr Paul Thomas surrendered his licence after being dragged through a legal quagmire by the Oregon health authorities for years over three solid and groundbreaking statistical vaccine studies conducted in his huge pediatric practice.

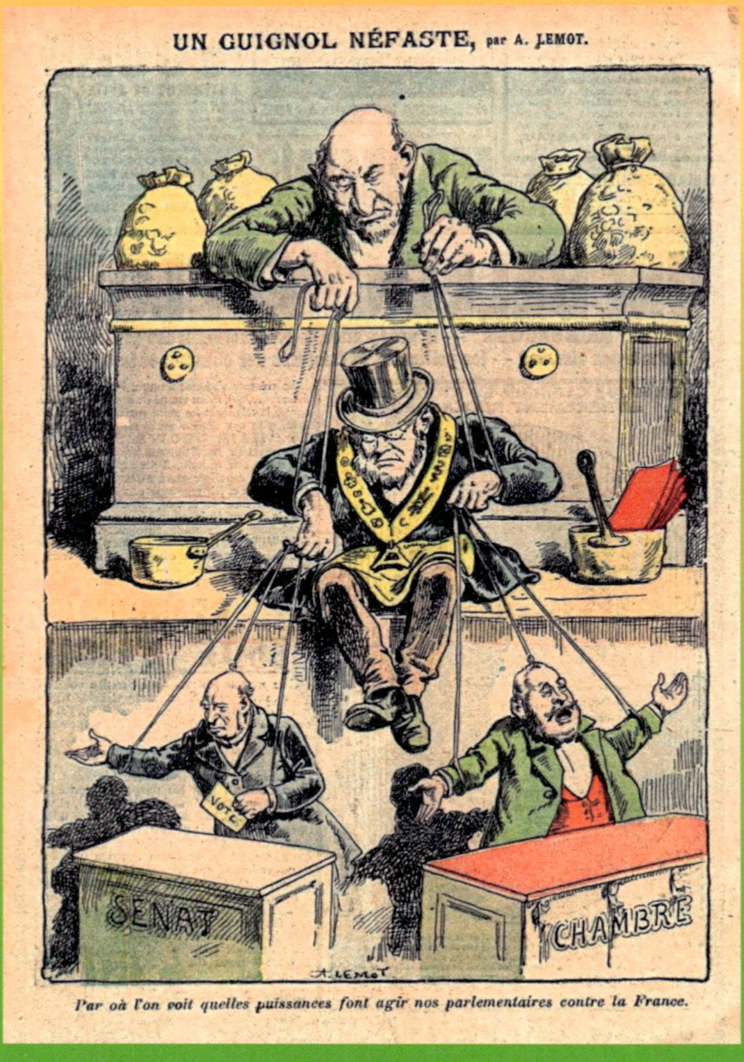

No words needed ...

Phasing out Microscopes?

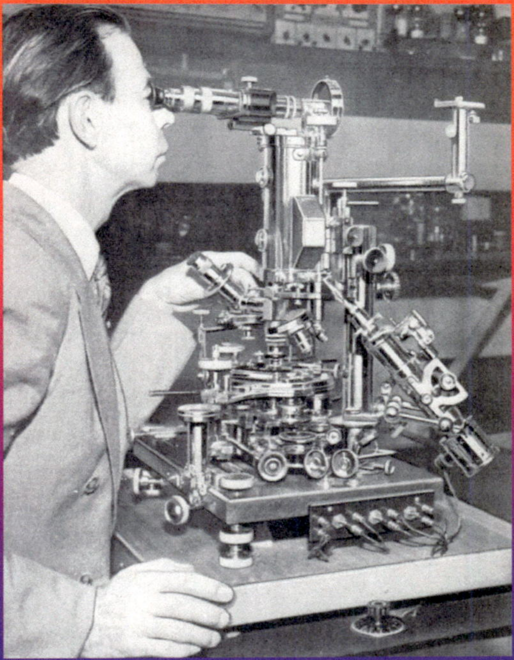

'Rife's Universal microscope had 5,000 moving parts, weighed 45 kilos and was ten times more powerful than any light source microscope that existed then or now.'
Steve Ross PhD. Rife Historian

There are three interesting facts I came across on my journey which seem unconnected until we piece them together.

Together they have helped to hide a world of contamination.

1. Royal Raymond Rife and the Universal Microscope

By 1933 Royal Raymond Rife had developed his Universal Microscope to the point where (we are told) it offered an optical magnification of living, moving, fluid organisms of 31,000 diameters from many angles. (There is controversy over these figures, and I wonder how one would measure the magnification potential of an instrument like this anyway?) Nevertheless, it was an incredible achievement. Fast forward to today and many optical microscopes, including those set up for live blood analysis, only magnify up to 4,000 diameters.

Electron microscopes offer much higher magnification than this, but the process tends to dry and kill live subjects such as parasites, cancer activity and blood contamination. Amazingly, Rife was able to highlight various elements of what he was seeing with different colours from the light spectrum itself.

> 'Every microbe, virus or bacterium glowed in its own unique colour.
> Cancer was in the ruby red spectrum.
> Typhus was blue.
> At this magnification there are worlds beyond worlds beyond worlds that we haven't even identified yet.'
> Royal Raymond Rife

He acquired and tuned a frequency machine to 60 different disease organisms, including leprosy, syphilis, sarcoma, bubonic plague, tetanus, strep, tuberculosis and cancer, so it could target and destroy microbes within diseased cells while leaving all the surrounding healthy cells intact. He was able to film this destruction happening in real time. Nearly a hundred years later this is still an amazing achievement.

ROYAL RAYMOND RIFE

The universal microscope, is the most powerful Rife scope, possessing a resolution of 31,000 diameters and magnification of 60,000 diameters. With this magnification it is possible to view the interior of the pin point cells situated between the normal tissue cells and just visible under the ordinary microscope.

We can even see the smaller cells which compose the interior of these pin-point cells.
When one of these smaller cells is magnified, still smaller cells are seen within it. When one of the still smaller cells is magnified, it too, is seen to be composed of even tinier cells.

ANNUAL REPORT
SMITHSONIAN INSTITUTION, 1944

Rife doesn't appear to be a boastful, money-hungry or fame seeking man. I tend to believe that his focus was always to use what he saw in his microscopes for the good of humanity.

Using these brilliant instruments for a medical study in the 1930s, Royal Raymond Rife cured every one of 14 terminal cancer patients within two months. It is one of the great tragedies of our time that in the following few years, this unassuming but brilliant scientist and his work were first celebrated as heroic, then destroyed in a nasty and complex tale of regulatory bullying, greed, deception and incompetence.

Sadly, even up to the present day, our research and medical history is littered with a very long list of people who have been sacked, stripped of their paper qualifications, persecuted, or worse for their life-giving discoveries, disclosure or ethics. We've already heard about Professor Chris Exley and Dr Paul Thomas, but, Dr Max Gerson, Dr Andrew Wakefield, Dr Stanislav Burzynski, Dr William Makis, Dr John Piesse, Dr Paul Marik, Dr Pierre Kory, Dr Suzanne Humphries, Dr Peter McCullough,

Dr James Thorpe, Dr Kevin Coleman, Dr David Nixon, Dr Andrew Katelaris, Dr My Le Trinh, Dr Paul Oosterhuis, Dr Andrew Moulden and Dr Jeff Bradstreet, spring to mind. There are many more.

The Universal microscope is no longer available to us but hopefully there are a few of these delicate and versatile instruments carefully hidden away somewhere waiting to be faithfully reproduced and nurtured back into existence.

It is now relatively easy to buy and use frequency machines which work on a similar principle and I believe we are finally in the dawn of acceptance of frequency medicine. Brain waves and heart beats are both electrical and it makes sense that specific electrical frequencies might be beneficial for them. (I comment more on this with a caution later in the book.)

How many millions of lives would have been saved if Royal Raymond Rife, the frequency machine and his magnificent Universal Microscope had been supported by the medical authorities, funded, protected, and marketed properly?

2. Medical Training: A big change in microscopic studies

Dr Lee Merritt (The Medical Rebel) recounts that when she first went to medical school in the 1970s, she was told that she wasn't a proper doctor unless she had a microscope in her clinic and used it on a daily basis to check a variety of biological samples such as blood, stools, urine and other samples. This is quick, cheap and confidential. It makes sense to me. Having your own microscope also means that you can easily see evidence of impurities in medications, anaesthetics, vaccines, food or water with your own eyes. Once you've seen contamination for yourself you can avoid it and sound the alarm to others.

She tells us that by the eighties, the very idea of having a working microscope in your clinic had been abandoned as old-fashioned and unnecessary. This means that doctors are no longer as in touch with what is really going on. When they send a sample off to the lab, there's no confidentiality and they usually see only figures and graphs when they come back.

It's not so easy to quietly check the purity of blood samples or mandated injections.

Does this mean that (unlike vets), as a profession they have become dependent on expensive lab reports, interpretation and possible manipulation, rather than their own perception, curiosity, experience and intuition?

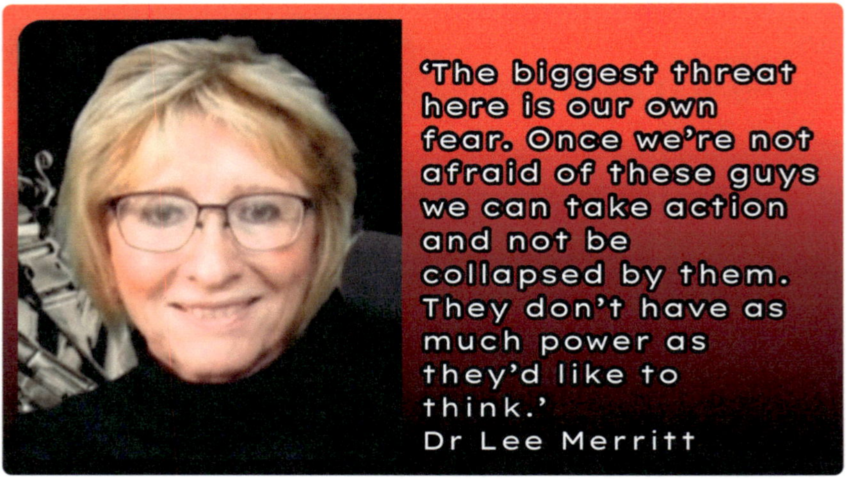

3. Live :lood Analysis

It's worth a few words here to explain the major difference between different types of microscopy.

Bright-field microscopy is fully lit from below. It's great for stained or coloured solid items and tissues, but living, transparent or unstained specimens usually look almost invisible.

Dark field microscopy is lit from the side like a spotlight and we might think of subjects such as our delicate little cells as stained glass windows which might look dim in normal light but which really stand out and sparkle against the darkness when light hits them at the right angle. What we see needs careful interpretation, but we can see a lot more with dark field.

Phase-contrast microscopy is excellent for seeing extra depth and detail inside unstained living cells and other structures.

Live blood analysis is the practice of examining fresh blood in dark field or phase contrast microscopy. We can see the cells and plasma clearly on an attached computer screen as it floats and swirls. The blood is ever-changing, but the condition of the cells reveals many secrets about the health of our bodies which are not easy to see with a normal microscope.

After having such a powerful and positive introduction to the idea of live blood analysis from Tony Robbins in 2004 and finding it easily available in a couple of clinics shortly afterwards, I was surprised to realise that when I came across it again twenty years later, that instead of flourishing as a valuable diagnostic tool, it had apparently fallen out of favour even in the field of natural medicine. It's regarded with suspicion as a pseudo-science and as something of a waste of time. Obviously, we need proper training and equipment standards for this technique but I believe this glimpse into the composition of living blood to be valuable. I think live blood checks are pretty much essential when contamination and frequencies are involved and anonymous aeroplanes are spraying unseen particles on us all.

These three historic observations lead us clearly to the elephant in the room.

The elephant in the room

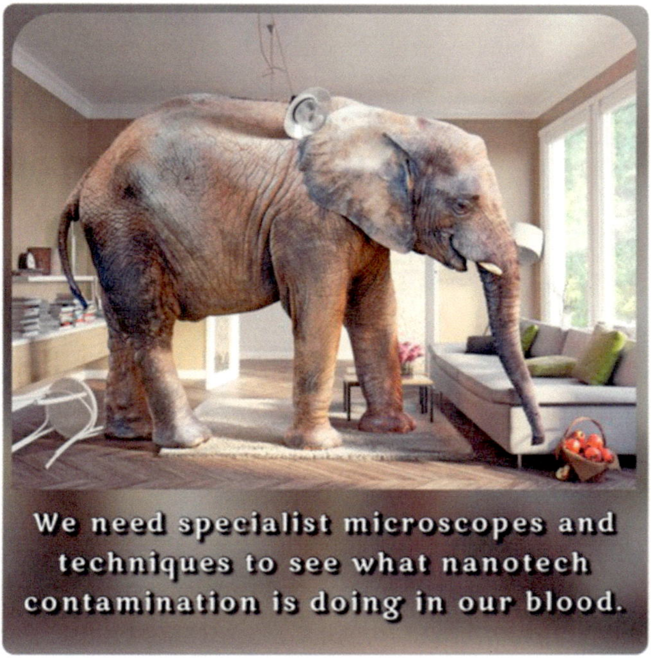

This contamination can increase, assemble, multiply and thicken our blood without us even knowing about it for months and years before it's a much bigger issue and physical problems show up. As with heart attacks and strokes, the first sign of trouble can be death.

From statements from Clifford Carnicom, Dr Ria Hayes, Dr Ana Milhacea, and others, it seems that if left unchecked, those nano-filaments, hydrogels and mesogens may form into bigger and bigger clumps until they form rubbery clots and fill vital veins and arteries.

Inventor Felipe Reitz adapted a thermography imaging machine to highlight blood clots in the body and is still discovering large blood clots running the length of veins and arteries, even in people showing no symptoms.

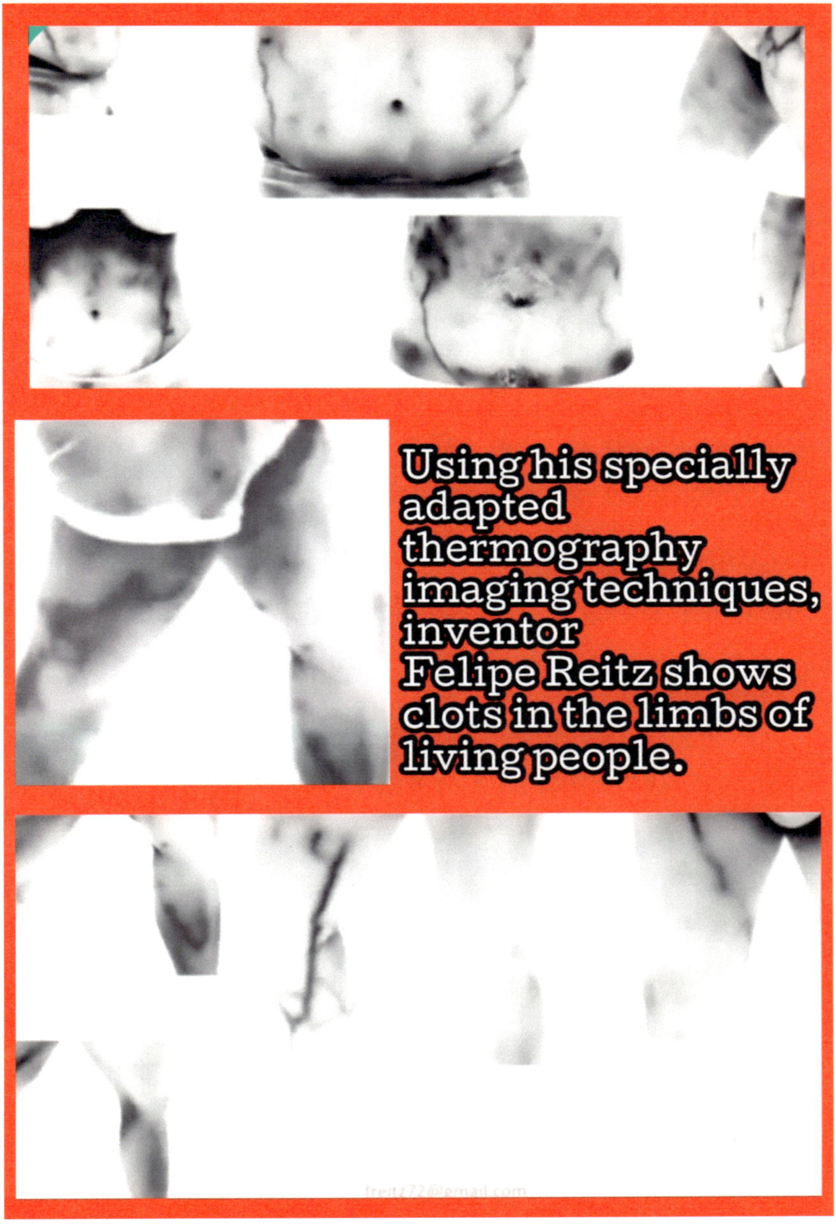
Using his specially adapted thermography imaging techniques, inventor Felipe Reitz shows clots in the limbs of living people.

John O'Looney

In 2022, John O'Looney, an honest, down-to-earth London undertaker and embalmer, first sounded the alarm about long, thick, rubbery 'calamari' type clots he was finding in the bodies he was embalming in the post covid shot era. US embalmer Richard Hirschman was finding the same clots and had the same courage to talk about them openly. Between them they had many decades of experience across the embalming and funeral industry and had never seen them before. These clots and so called 'coffee grounds' micro-clots were blocking up both veins and arteries of otherwise healthy young bodies. These were described in Ed Dowd's book originally published in October 2022. 'Cause Unknown'.

There is even a term for these deaths: Sudden Adult Death syndrome or SADs. They couldn't be sadder.

An international survey of embalmers was conducted by retired Major Tom Haviland in mid 2025. A questionnaire filled in and returned by approximately 200 embalmers from around the world confirmed that they were still seeing these new clots in around 20% of bodies.

There are many images and clips of these rubbery clots stuffed into vials like big rubber bands. We also have clips of these long stringy clots being pulled out of the veins and arteries of living patients during dialysis-type EBOO treatments. I even have a rubbery clot of my very own.

More on this later.

Coroners, pathologists and police who should be investigating this are often quiet. It used to be standard practice for full autopsies to be done on all unexpected deaths to rule out foul play. John O'Looney tells us that since 2022 this is not always the case. A previously healthy young person can die in their sleep or drop dead in the kitchen and no-one in authority bothers to find out why. Coroners are silent about this. Retired Major Tom Haviland tells us that surgeons removing these new clots from living patients will routinely throw them away rather than have them examined by pathology labs to see what they are or how to prevent them.

Universities in Australia, the U.S. and the U.K. fearful of their funding, are so far showing little to no interest in studying this phenomenon.

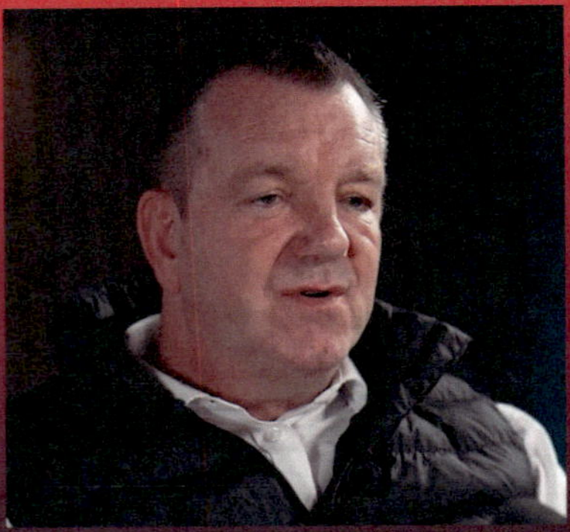

'I'll keep shouting about these rubbery clots. If it costs me my life, I'll go to my maker with a clear conscience.'
John O'Looney,
Embalmer and
Funeral Director

Rubbery clots

If we can't see the inner workings of our live blood, I believe that in 2026 we have to assume that the vast majority of us are affected by this new contamination. It's my belief that at this stage in our development as a species, we have to open ourselves to remedies that work, especially when alternatives are few and far between.

If I could suggest that you rock up to your friendly local nanotech detox practitioner for some supplements and procedures to clear up the problem, solving this mystery and avoiding injury would be a lot easier. As at early 2026, there are probably less than 50 clinics specialising in these issues around the world. Other answers are available to us to keep this clotting under control and I am more optimistic now than I was when I first started writing.

However, as at May 2026, turning up at virtually any clinic anywhere and expecting them to know anything about this new contamination in our blood is like turning up at our local Ford dealership and hoping they can fix our flying saucer.

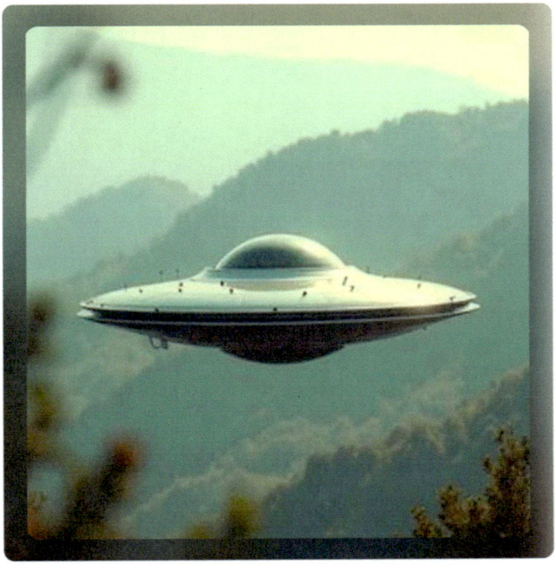

We have to become our own detectives and our own healers here, using our faith, intuition and common sense, working alongside trusted and trusting naturopaths, homeopaths and even the occasional open-minded doctor to solve the mystery and discover solutions that work for us.

We're all going to have to educate ourselves together. We need to keep our intuition sharp and our wits about us.

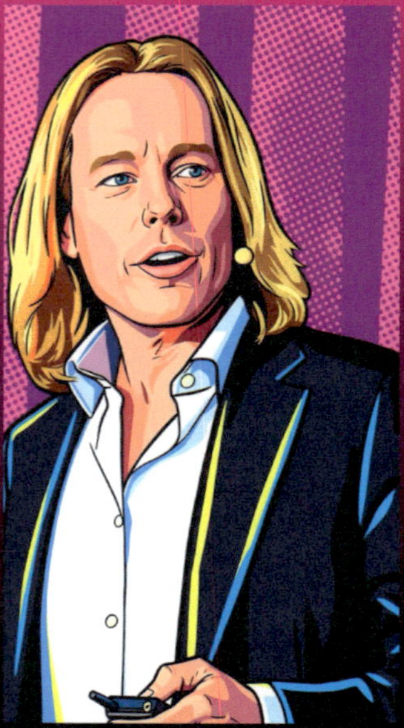

'Right now we've got to think outside the box. They're using the metals as antenna. If they're using synthetic stuff we might have to use synthetic stuff as well. We've got to get the metals out of the system.'
Dr Ed Group DC. ND

Unchartered Territory

Real scientific breakthrough and medical insights don't arrive fully fledged with big studies and fanfares. Real discovery presents itself to the open minded with tiny hints, clues and questions. They may be seen in miniscule changes on a microscope slide or half-whispered by patients whose health professional actually listens to them.

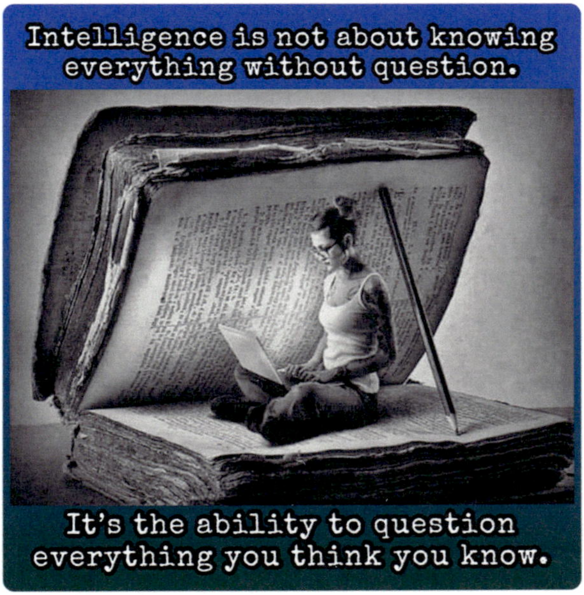

Practitioners and researchers who assume they know everything shut themselves off to these subtle hints of new discovery. They can cost lives and hold the process back for decades. Maybe this is where we are with these unnerving filaments, clots and cancers. I personally feel the urgency of this work to put together a range of possible solutions and starter points for further exploration as best I can.

Inner Guidance

Before we look at what these nano filaments are, I want to make it clear that because this journey is so new, a small amount of the information I share has been acquired with the help of my own muscle testing, a kinesiologist and a psychic reader. I usually indicate this by the phrase 'I believe …'

If you prefer not to accept the reality of this guidance, no worries, just skip the bits you don't like and meet me on the other side ….

I hope this situation will change fairly quickly as word spreads and people share information, but for now I believe we need all the intuition and psychic guidance we can get.

My family was never religious but my mother used to say that 'God is within us'. I heard this without thinking about it too much, but as life progresses, I understand the truth of it more and more. Wayne Dyer wisely told us to be as Christ-like or Buddha-like as we could and many of us in these strange times feel called to serve humanity in various ways. As Bob Proctor used to ask: 'How is God to work except through our hands?'

We can often sense if someone or some thing is genuine or not and I believe that our individual journey through this strange situation is often going to be guided by our higher selves.

Just as a good tree bears good fruit, good people work to serve others and the world around them. Some people are doing the opposite and it is by their actions, rather than their words that we can tell if they are serving humanity or not.

As the old truism goes, 'Actions speak louder than words.'

As Jesus is quoted as saying: ‘By their fruits shall ye know them.’

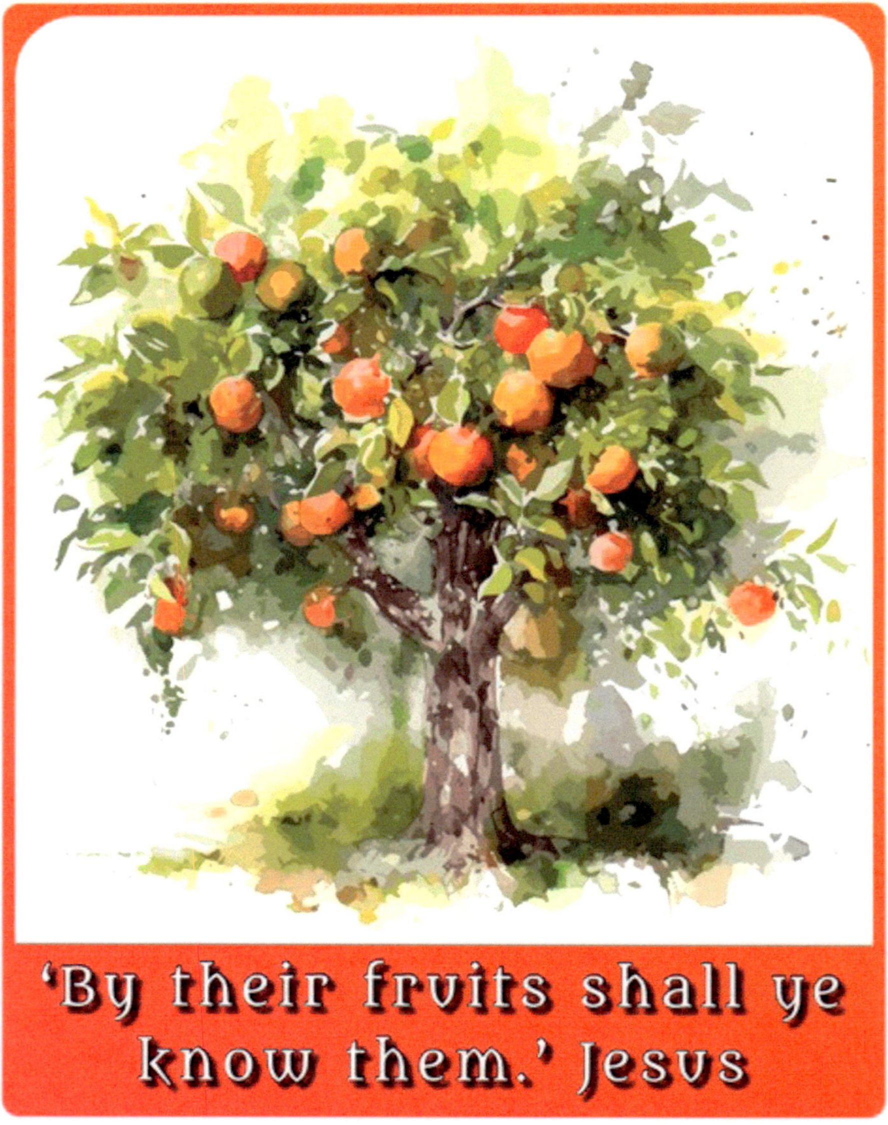

Higher self

We are spiritual beings, tiny slivers of the God energy.

Who better to give us guidance than an (almost) all knowing part of ourselves? Before we go any further, I'm going to describe three ways of contacting our higher selves. For many people their connection with the divine may be through prayer, and meditation. I'm going to focus here on the slightly more unusual muscle testing, kinesiology and using a genuine psychic reader.

I'll start with muscle testing as it's the simplest and the most easily accessible to everyone.

Muscle Testing

Muscle testing is a switch to our intuition. I've been doing it for years to guide me through life in various ways. We all understand intuition or 'gut feel'. Many of us have looked at new homes for the first time and know the feeling of 'Yes!' as we walked through the door. Many of us recognise times when we made bad decisions - hooking up with the wrong person or signing the wrong document while our stomach was churning, our hands were sweaty with anxiety or we just had an uneasy feeling that something wasn't right. Once we have a switch to those feelings and faith in that intuition, we can be more aware of what a good decision feels like. That way we can hopefully avoid those mistakes as soon as we see them on the horizon.

Kinesiologists use this incredible resource in a more highly tuned way to help the body, which we'll come to later, but I learned muscle testing from the teachings of Dr David Hawkins. I read his book 'Power vs Force' in around 2007 and one sentence imprinted itself in my brain:

'You can muscle test for Universal Truth'
Dr David Hawkins

Those words stayed with me for years until I chanced upon some of his DVDs and learned enough to develop my own muscle testing technique which I have used ever since. People who use a pendulum or read Tarot cards for good are also tapping into this same energy.

When we hear a statement of truth: 'It's a sunny day' or 'I am sitting outside' our body responds with strength. Our muscles are strong without us even realising and if someone presses our arm or we use our hands to test ourselves while we hold that thought, we are firm and solid.

If we were to sit outside in the sunshine and say, 'It's pouring with rain,' our muscles would become as weak as a baby without us even realising. We would have little strength to resist our own self-testing or someone pressing on our arm.

I wouldn't bet my house on it, but we can also test for, say, taking a new job, moving house, starting or ending a relationship, or going on a trip. We might say, 'It's in my best and highest interest to take this new job with Smith Brothers.'

'It's in my best and highest interest to visit Sydney this month.' 'This relationship is right for me.' These are things we don't know yet and some we could never know. I frequently use muscle testing in my writing. For example, I often muscle test what percentage of you wonderful readers are able to understand a particular word, phrase, or piece of information.

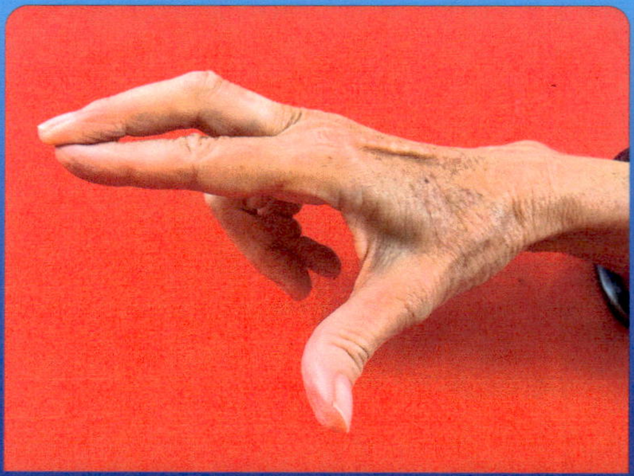

Single hand muscle testing

So how is it done? Assuming you don't have a willing partner with you at all times, you'll need to self-test. The most subtle test is to press the index finger and middle finger of the same hand against each other a bit as if you were crossing your fingers (probably the non-dominant hand would be best). This one is a bit too subtle for me but it's handy to do in secret during meetings or interviews.

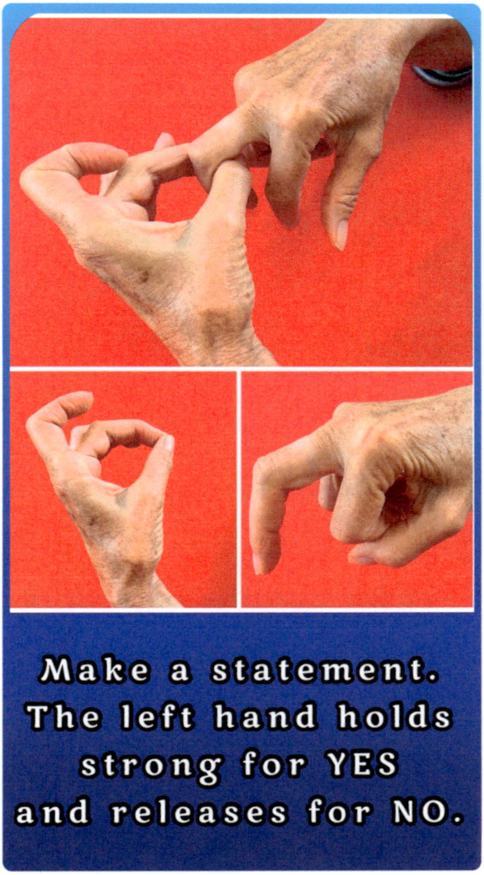

I use both hands. I make a loop between the middle finger and thumb of my left hand so this is the switch, and I bend the middle finger of my other hand to make the hook. This is not quite as easy to hide as the first muscle test but a bit easier to learn. Have a play with this and find a switch you like.

I even muscle-test on the steering wheel if I want to test something and I'm driving on quieter roads.

We should always make a statement, not a question. If it's true, the switch will stay strong. (This isn't a test of strength. We might use the same amount of force we might use to flick an actual light switch). If it's not true it will release at once.

Occasionally our responses can get confused and we can reset them. Just leaving a subject for a while and coming back to it can give us more clarity. We can also, believe it or not, reset by thumping our chest at the start of the session a bit like Tarzan or his gorilla friends might. This is called the thymus thump and apparently it releases fear, increases the life force energy we are working with, increases strength and vitality, and boosts your immune system. Who knew?

Practicing this wonderful new skill at your fingertips is key. There are only a few rules to remember:

- Find a peaceful space without background distractions.
- Always work with a statement, not a question.
- Speak your statements out loud for clarity.
- Start off with a few statements you know the answers to.
- Keep a detached, mildly interested perspective.

If the statement being tested is so important to you that you're attached to the answer: 'I'm pregnant,' or 'I've got the job,' for example, you may not get an accurate reading. You may need to find an objective friend or reader to test on your behalf.

They may be many kilometres away. Distance is not important to this process as long as the person testing is clear on the question.

You can test for whether your body needs a food or supplement or not. I do this with almost every supplement I take. I hold the bottle close to my cheek or even just put my hand on a food in the wholefoods market and test: 'This is good for me today.' The answer usually comes up clearly. I love fresh berries and always test these to find the ones that are relatively pesticide free and healthy to eat. (Spoiler alert: fast foods, fries and coke aren't going to test positive any time soon.)

When checking percentages, say, for example 'The percentage of people who enjoyed the talk I gave is …' (start low) over 50%, (test yes) over 60%, (test yes) over 70%, (test no). This means your final answer is between 60% and 70%. Now fine-tune the exact number: 'Over 61% (test yes) over 62% (test yes) over 63% (test no).' This means that your final answer is that 63% of the people enjoyed your talk. Once you get the hang of this, it's very easy.

I test people's calibration in a similar way. This is my own definition of calibration based on Dr David Hawkins' scale of human enlightenment from 1-1000. I don't agree with most of his results on this but the scale starts at 1, which is the worst sort of soulless being and goes up to Jesus Christ at 1,000, followed by a very small group of enlightened masters like, say, the Buddha. A balanced, enlightened person will calibrate much higher than say, a belligerent criminal. I have found that this measurement usually holds steady, like our character, or the climate. I believe it indicates the amount of light we hold as an individual soul in human form. We are all on our soul's individual journey. When you meet someone for the first time and get on with them easily as if you've known them for ever, it's highly likely that you are calibrating on a similar level.

I'll keep this fairly general, but when I first learned this technique ten years ago, I calibrated everyone I could think of in a long list. Since then I have found that most of humanity has gone up about 50 points on this list of 1-1,000. I *personally* get that most human beings are now over 600. Unfortunately, some people's life choices, and lack of integrity have brought their calibration way down to the point, I believe, that the soul has left.

What I think of as frequency is more changeable from hour to hour, a bit like the weather. Getting an unexpected bill or finding that the dog has chewed our new shoes can bring our frequency down a bit. On the other hand, We may meet up with a friend or get a lovely compliment to lift our mood again. It's important that we pay attention to our frequency and learn how to 'lift our spirits' quickly ourselves. I have to do this occasionally when writing about these dark subjects. It could easily be depressing, but I seem to be built for this, and a walk in our lovely nearby countryside is plenty to get me back on track.

I wouldn't necessarily trust muscle testing with everything, but I use it to guide me as I might use the well-meaning words of a wise friend to navigate through a challenging time.

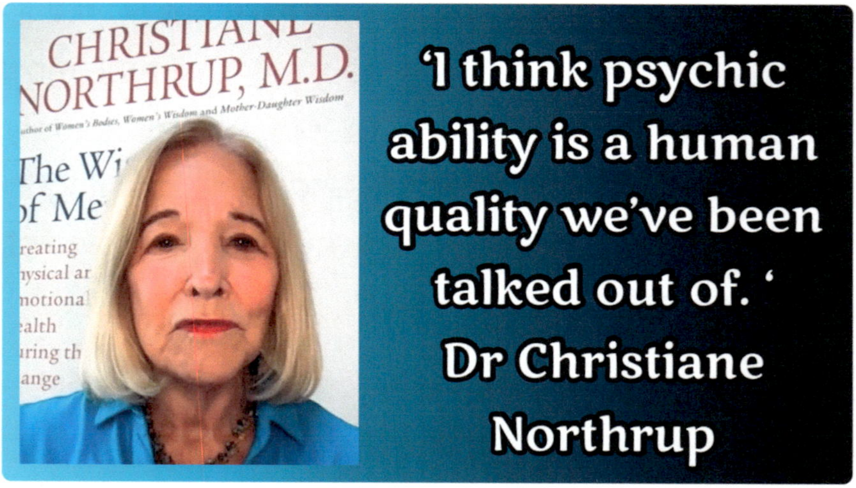

Kinesiology

Kinesiologists take the skill of simple muscle testing to a whole new level and work with our higher selves and our physical bodies in a variety of ways to tell us exactly what is happening with us in body, mind, and spirit. They can then recommend the foods, supplements, and lifestyle changes we need to find our way back to health.

Kinesiology is especially important when we know something isn't right, but we're not sure what it is or how to treat it. It's great to check which supplements or medication your body needs. A modality like this which works with energy is also good to cross-check your own muscle testing or psychic readings to improve accuracy and confidence.

I believe kinesiologists and psychics are essential to help us get out of this nano-filament fairy-lights situation. As we stand in 2026, there are probably still less than a couple of hundred professionals around the world who acknowledge what's happening or who have any idea how to resolve it.

Psychic Reading

The beauty of a psychic reader is that in my case she, like the kinesiologist, provides a cross-reference and back up for my own intuition and muscle testing. I seem to be designed emotionally tough enough to stand my ground when writing or speaking uncomfortable truths. In the ten years I've been visiting my friend and psychic reader I've learned that she sees and senses far more than I do about important aspects of my life. I am blessed to have a group of other-worldly beings who, although they certainly don't write for me, guide my writing and send information and extraordinary synchronicities my way from time to time. The psychic reading is often more about the overview, while the kinesiologist is more about the physical detail, although there is overlap.

Chemtrails

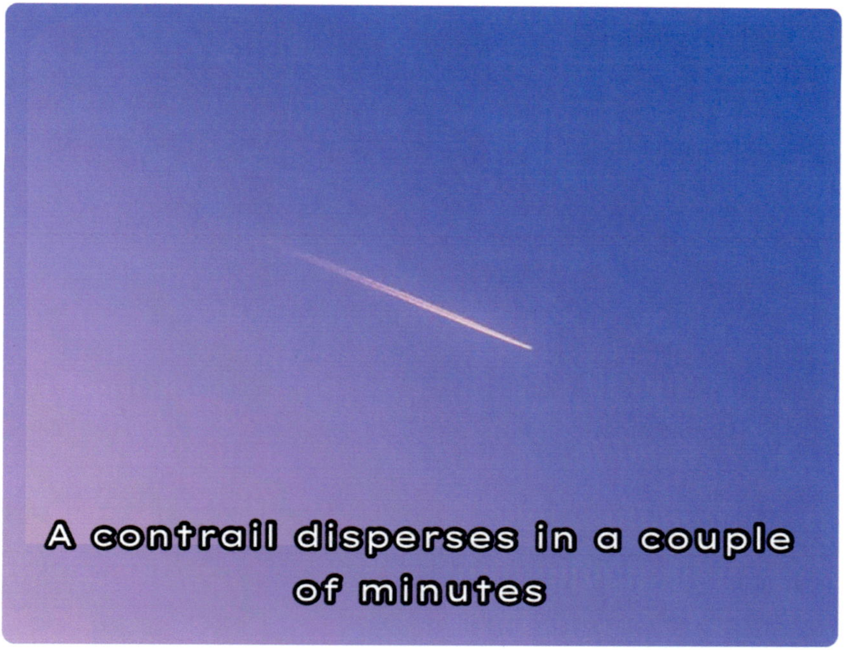

I know a little about chemtrails. When I was a child, we lived underneath one of the flight paths from what was then Ringway Airport and is now Manchester International Airport. We were so close that we couldn't hear ourselves talk for a minute or so while the 'planes went over and on a sunny day we could watch aeroplanes from elsewhere high in the sky in the same flight path, their white contrails behind them shining in the clear blue skies for a few brief moments before they disappeared into nothing.

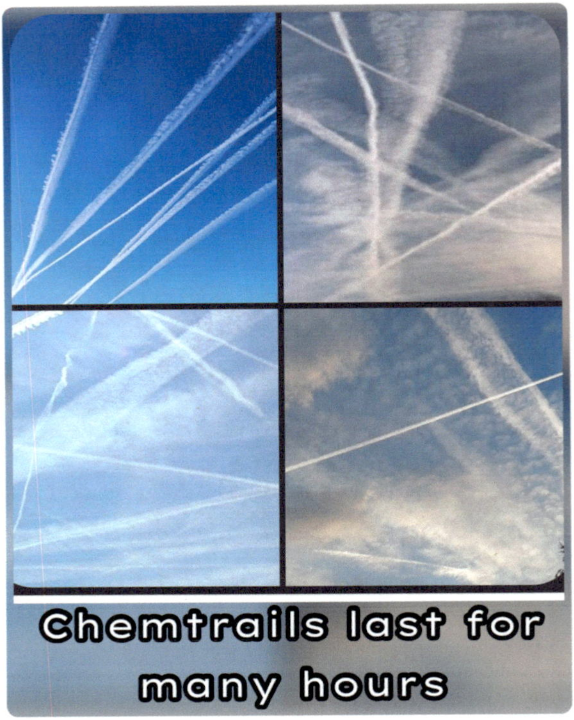

According to Clifford Carnicom, since around the year 1999 we have seen increasing numbers of chemtrails in our skies. They follow ‘planes like contrails but linger for hours and days, causing thick, hazy checks and stripes in our clear blue skies. We can often see them spreading out until the whole sky is grey and overcast.

They seem to come mostly from a random collection of specially adapted planes flown by mercenaries with little or no conscience. For anyone thinking that these are being sprayed from normal commercial flights, it's interesting to note that normal flights, like buses, follow a regular daily or weekly schedule and yet we can see for ourselves that one day the sky looks clear and sunny while the next day it can be completely covered in a checkerboard of lingering trails.

These chemtrails are no secret. It dawned on me recently that a whole generation of has grown to adulthood thinking that this is normal. These are not normal. Many of us have been seeing them for years. As at early 2026, eleven US states have held hearings to prohibit or criminalize geo-engineering and weather modification. Apart from injections, I believe this is how most of the toxins are spread to us all. This is often called cloud-seeding or geo-engineering, as it seems to manipulate our weather, but in a smaller circle of researchers including the Carnicom Institute, it's also known as bio-engineering.

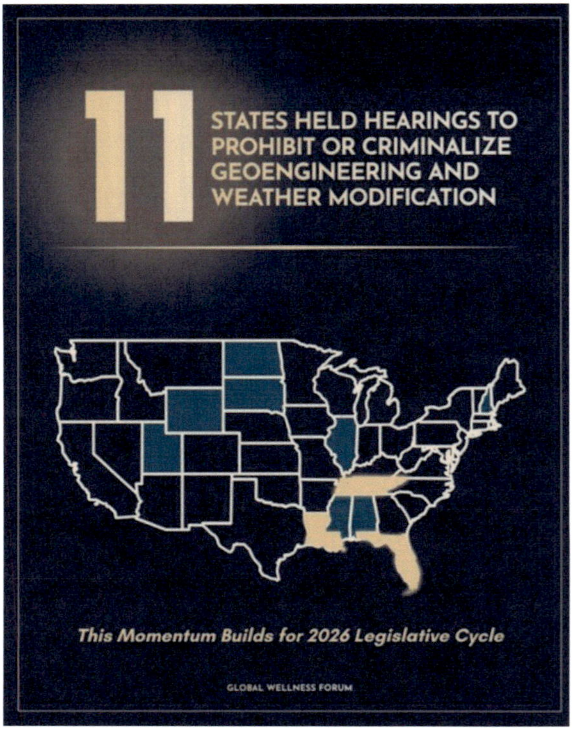

I make it a rule not to worry too much about things I can do nothing about, so until my first shocking live blood analysis, I hadn't given chemtrails much thought. I didn't like them, but I wasn't concerned that they were doing me any harm.

However, these chemtrails are made up of a variety of toxic cocktails, nano-particles and synthetic biology which assembles and adds to the contaminants in our blood. Some contaminants first appeared with the covid shots in 2021. Some of them are caused by shedding from one person to another, but now in 2026, I believe most of them are being sprayed on us from the skies. We are now truly all in this together.

We don't need to delve too deeply here into who's poisoning us from every angle or why. That's the necessary job of dedicated people like Elana Freeland who has documented this in detail for over a decade. Or Sabrina Wallace, who has inside information on many programs. It's a deep, dark hole. I'm just going to list some of their toxins from some of these programs together. Some of them I've known about for decades. Some of them I've only heard about in the last few months.

Chemtrails: aluminium, barium, strontium, cadmium, cesium, lithium, titanium. Other poisons: glyphosate, mercury, aluminium, fluoride, vaccines, covid, spike proteins: natural and synthetic parasites, graphene oxide: nano-flaments, self-assembling hydrogels: rubbery clots, moulds: electro-magnetic frequencies, directed energy weapons: genetically weaponised pathogens, bacteria, yeasts and a variety of deadly artificial snake, spider and cone snail venoms from around the world.

Some I didn't believe myself at first, but I've listened to enough detailed conversations and seen enough in my own blood to come to my own conclusion that these toxins are real. They are often unnoticed and unacknowledged, invasive, multiplying and possibly deadly.

Nasty as all this is, Dr Ed Group tells us that the biggest threats to our health and wellbeing are still:

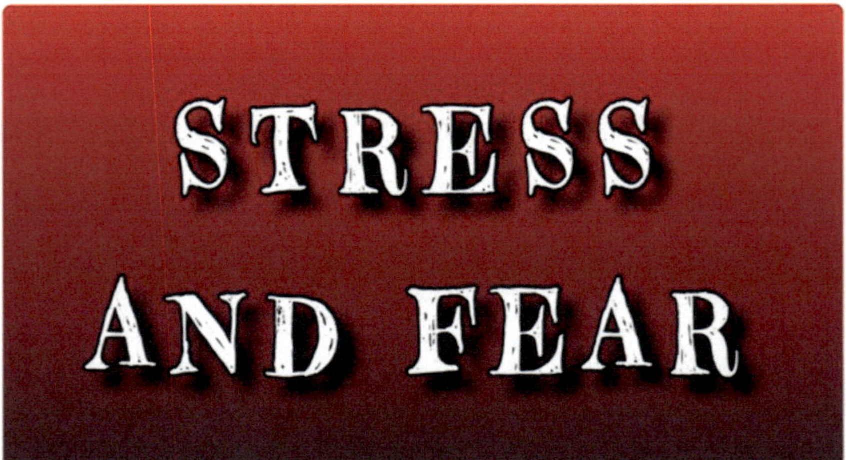

The very reason I'm writing this book at all is that we now have some remedies to keep these nasties at bay.

On the plus side, I truly believe that those of us who work for the benefit of humanity in various ways have God on our side. We're smart, we're savvy, and we're incredibly resilient. Once we decide what action to take, we can lift ourselves out of fear and empower ourselves.

There seem to be three main camps in this exploration:

Self-assembling nano-filaments, genetically modified viruses and various venoms.

I believe there is some overlap.

Nano-Filaments

I believe that the nano-filaments assembling in my own blood were from chemtrails, but because they've been sprayed over everything they may also be picked up from water, food, air, vaccines, medications, shedding from some vaccinated people, blood transfusions and dental anaesthetics. They appear to be intelligent and self-assemble in the blood creating micro-sized structures bigger than red blood cells and big enough for us to see under the microscope.

They have shown themselves in our lakes, rivers and grasslands, snow, fog and flood waters as well as in our own urine, blood, sweat and tears. Nano-sized toxins are more damaging to the body than micro-sized ones. They penetrate everywhere, crossing cell membranes and the blood-brain barrier, and because they are smaller they have a larger surface area to interact with the body.

It's not only us, unfortunately. According to Ana Milhacea and her colleagues around the world, these things are found in grass-fed meat and even in the blood of wild animals like deer, rabbits and squirrels. I've been told that even remote farmland in Australia has been contaminated with aluminium and other toxic metals thought to have come from chemtrails.

After input from a handful of scientists, the psychic and the kinesiologist in different sessions, as well as my own muscle testing, we came to a number of conclusions which we all largely agree on:

Over 90% of the Australian people have these nano-micro filaments in their blood.

As far as I can tell, the nano-micro filaments may be a first stage of the contamination and exposure to some EMFs activates them in some way so that they clump together. We might think of this like a lump of hair gel that sits in our blood making it 'sticky'. It has a tendency to grow on its own, it may respond to heat, and may develop into rubbery clots or more nano-micro filaments. Whatever it is, it's certainly not something we want gumming up our blood or our organs.

This contamination seems to dull the negative electrical charge of the blood which causes the blood cells to clump together. It reduces the amount of oxygen they carry, prevents detoxing and causes the body to be more susceptible to EMFs, Wifi and cancers.

Morgellons Fibres

We can see Morgellons-like fibres on our clothes and even under our skin with a violet-light scope a bit like the sort we used to love in night clubs and discos.

These fibres are different from normal polyester fibres that you might pick up from the air, your furnishings or carpets. According to an experienced microscopist, they don't burn and often assemble themselves into continuous threads when placed near each other.

Under the skin these same fibres can be seen with the skin scope as fluorescent spots which are often itchy and quite knotted together. They can form open wounds that won't heal. We do have a couple of answers for these among our remedies.

We can be cautious, but we can't escape these things without ruining our lives in the process.

We need to join forces and take on this challenge together.

> It's not a choice to stand by and hope that this is all going to be ok.
> You have to do something to clear them.
> Your body needs a partner in all this.'
> Maria Crister. Abeytu Naturals

Genetically Modified Pathogens

There appears to be an overlap or contradiction between the following research and the proven existence of of nano and micro-filaments in blood, urine, anaesthetics and other medications.

As a lay person, I believe both avenues of research to be valid and I suspect that they might run side by side. We're going to have to live with that contradiction for now, and It doesn't change the direction of our main quest … How do we get rid of whatever might be clogging up our veins and arteries?

'So far today I've embalmed two bodies and one of them was full of these clots. If people think this is over, it's not.'
Richard Hirschman
Embalmer
September 2025

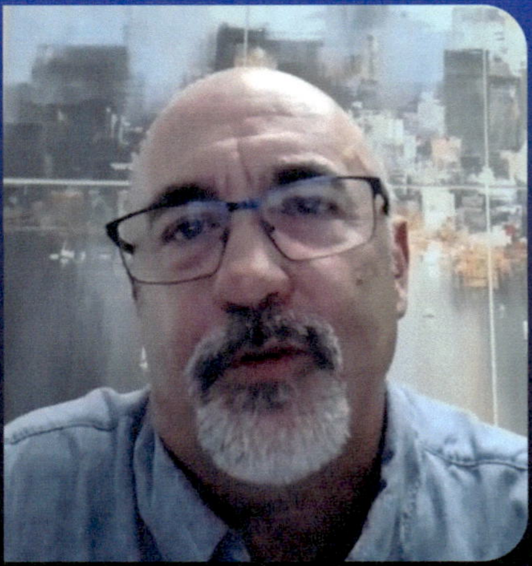

In August 2025, the Reese Report carried a detailed and referenced interview with independent lead scientist Greg Harrison and Tom Haviland about some of the biological processes involved in the formation of these white fibrous clots.

Then we had a second on-line symposium on the SGT Report: 'Documenting Genocide,' with Todd Callender, embalmer Richard Hirschman, Tom Haviland, Greg Harrison, Dr Sherri Tenpenny, Dr Rima Laibow and Dr Bill Lionberger

https://www.bitchute.com/video/8oTqkjmpJQfo/.

It was great to have confirmation by impeccably ethical names of long standing like Dr Sherri Tenpenny and Dr Rima Laibow that this is a real issue. They both commended Greg Harrison's in-depth research.

'Ralph Baric is a leading coronavirus expert who spent decades engineering chimeric (genetically modified) viruses in collaboration with China.
Peter Dasik, Head of the Eco Health Alliance, funnelled millions of American taxpayer dollars into this research.' Anon

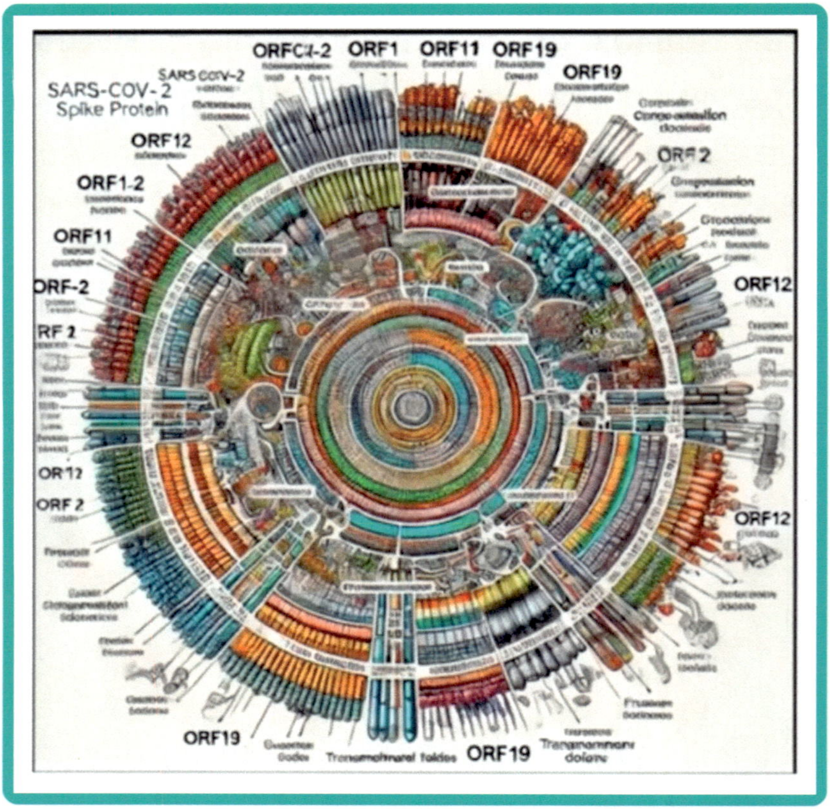

So, what are these strange ORFs? In a virus, an ORF is an open reading frame and it works like this: If we bake a cake, we might think about the ingredients we want to use. We have the basic flour, eggs, butter and sugar but we might add lemon, nuts, cinnamon or chocolate to vary the flavours. These extra additions are like the ORFs.

> 'The white rubbery clots being found globally by embalmers are real. They are not rare and sadly they are becoming common. They were not seen before 2021.'
>
> Greg Harrison,
> Retired Organic Chemist

These people seem to have been doing the same thing with viruses, except they have been selecting ORFs from a witches' brew of 'gain of function' effects such as higher infection rates, increased clotting or bleeding, skin issues, breathing issues or destruction of the immune system. They appear to have chosen these features from a selection of the nastiest infections and poisons on the planet, think ebola, marburg, zika, lassa, plague and smallpox. All sliced and diced into specially modified viruses to make us as sick as possible.

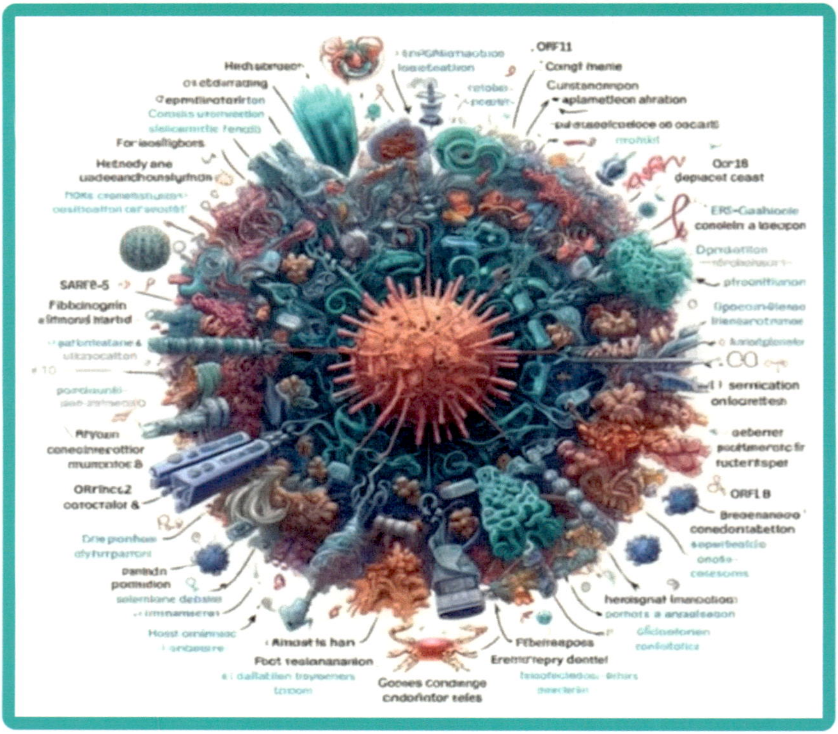

Retired organic chemist Greg Harrison tells us that a large university helped with some of his research under the strict ruling that they would never be identified. Such is the fear, censorship and control surrounding these issues.

The amyloid proteins seem to begin as micro clots or 'coffee grounds' clots. They are abnormal fibrin-based misfolded proteins. Once an amyloid is misfolded, the body can't deal with it and it grows.

We might have heard of amyloid plaques in the brain in Alzheimer's and Parkinson's disease but now apparently it can be found throughout the body in veins and arteries. Greg takes us meticulously through dozens of scientific papers backing up his research. All this is too much for casual listeners, but this body of work could be one of the starting points for universities, hospitals and institutions funded by our taxpayer dollars to use as a basis for research to find answers.

> 'No matter the obstacles we face – whether physical, mental, emotional, or genetic – our brains and bodies are designed to adapt, heal, and thrive.'
> Dr Ed Group

Here is more research from New Zealand on what these clots may be:

'The elemental data confirms it's not just protein; the clots are a hybrid material our bodies are forced to make but not equipped to clear.'
Dr Bruce Rapley and Dr Matt Shelton,

New Zealand Doctors Speaking Out With Science https://nzdsos.com

https://nzdsos.com/2026/02/04/breaking-research-decodes-the-mystery-of-the-rubbery-white-clots

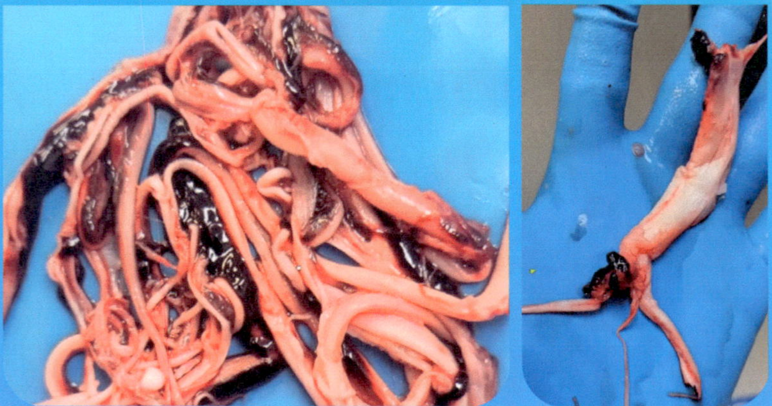

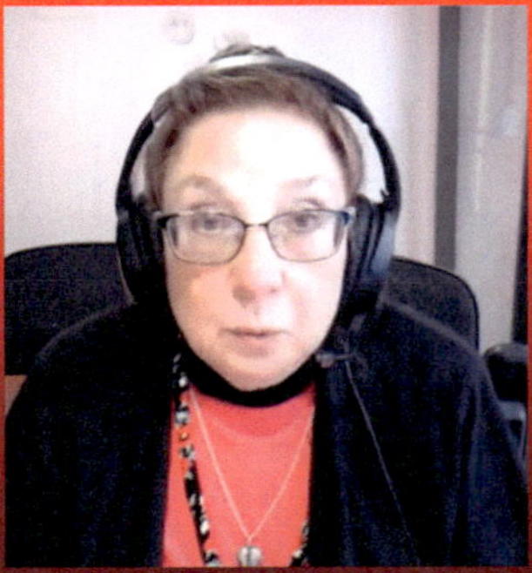

'EMF frequencies interact with phosphorus. Could it be possible that some of these unusual 'planking' deaths are being triggered by invisible signals?'
Dr Rima Laibow.

Greg Harrison and his team found that these clots have around nine times the amount of phosphorous of normal clots. The research papers state that when phosphorous binds with our proteins it forms new chemical entities that do not resemble any natural amino acids. This leads to disease. (I now believe that low zeta potential causing the red blood cells to clump may be a key factor in all this.)

'I began noticing a change in the blood around 2022. Strange filaments and unusual globular formations I had never seen before. At first I dismissed them as random anomalies or artefacts, but over time they became increasingly common and are now present in everyone I examine, regardless of age or vaccination status. They are even in children.'

Kirsty Bednar BHSc(Comp Med), ND.

Venoms

When we think of snake venom, we think of people painstakingly 'milking' the fangs of a deadly snake into a glass beaker and ending up with a few drops.

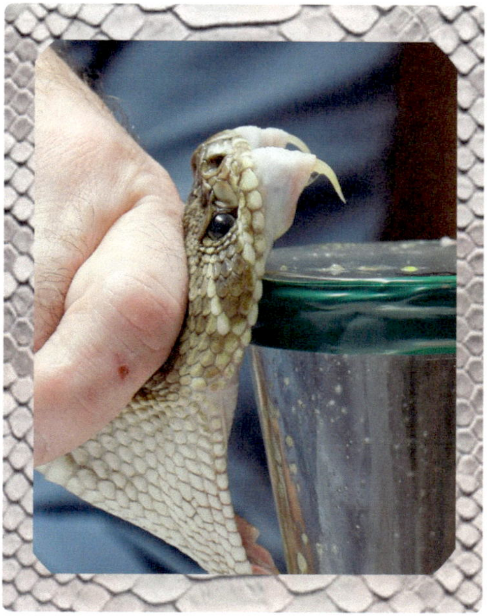

Horrifying though it is, we now know that artificial snake and snail venoms are manufactured in large quantities. These venomous cocktails target the nicotine receptors. (When I checked this with my psychic reader friend, the poor woman confirmed it with uncontrollable gagging.)

According to Bryan Ardis, it appears that many companies had combined various toxins from 36 deadly snake and snail venoms from around the world. They reproduced them in the lab, and manufactured a selection of them in random batches.

Did they inject them into millions of innocent arms?

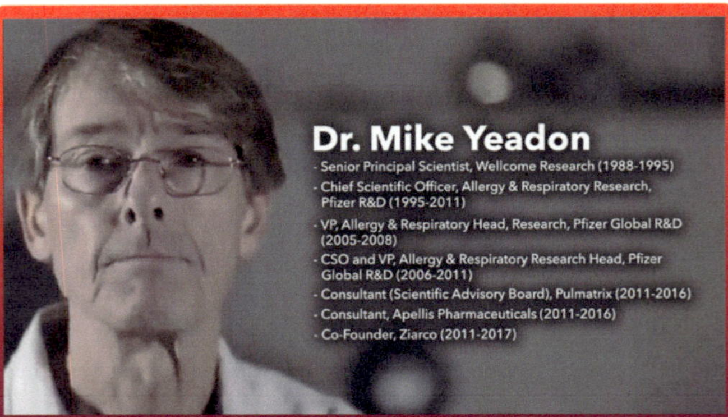

'VAERS (Vaccine Adverse Events Reporting System) reports have to include a verified batch number and batches have up to 1.5 million vials in them. Some have nearly 6,000 adverse reactions, then it drops down suddenly to under 5 in other batches. This is clearly not the same product. Vaccine companies would know about this. It's not an accident.'

We have known for a number of years now that the covid shot batches varied wildly, with some being more lethal than others.

The huge variety of 'side' effects may have been due to different combinations of venom. I wonder if some of those sneaky ORFS had anything to do with snake venoms?

This industry has a name. It's called venomics. Research like this is often claimed to be therapeutic. Some may indeed be of use for those suffering from actual snake bites, but statements like this from the industry itself suggest that we should pay close attention to their fascination with deadly poisons:

> The application of synthetic biology to venom research can achieve great advances in the understanding and utilization of the deadliest weapons found in the animal kingdom.
> PMID 37207126

Apparently, if we are bitten by a poisonous snake in real life, even if we have an antidote quickly and recover, we can suffer some effects from the poisoning for years to come.

I still hold the faith that many people had saline shots.

I don't believe that these three assaults on the health and wellbeing of ourselves, animals and Mother Earth herself are mutually exclusive. I believe they all add up to the bigger picture which, as at 2026, is still being ignored by our institutions.

> If you want to find the secrets of the universe, think in terms of energy, frequency and vibration.
>
> Nikola Tesla

Rescuing Ourselves

I wrote about Joe Dispenza's original story of miraculous healing in my last book, 'Detox After Covid and Thrive' and I'm including him here front and centre. The work he has been doing with his team for many years is profound, ground breaking and scientifically verified. Many of the thousands of people attending his seminars come for healing and transformation. He has helped these people rewire the way they think, feel, and heal. As he tells us, 'Your thoughts can make you sick, but your thoughts can also make you well.'

I don't believe faith is the whole answer to what we face now, but I certainly believe it can help.

He suggests that we get really clear on what we want by asking ourselves questions which demand descriptive answers. We need to create images so clear we can step into them, so our brain is not an unwitting record anchoring us to a past we didn't want, but a convincing map of the future.

We can't resolve a problem from the past. We have to free ourselves by disconnecting and moving beyond it.

Maybe it's like unhooking the heavy burden of our limiting beliefs from our beautiful physical vehicle and becoming, as he says: 'No-body, no-one, no-where, and no-time.' This is the space we can create from.

> **'The mind and body are intimately connected, and what we think and feel affects every cell in our body.'**
> **Dr Joe Dispenza**

I feel that this faith is the foundation of any healing suggestions or protocols we might choose.

Pictures and words are important for this creation. Years ago many of us cut pictures out of magazines to make life maps of the lives we wanted on big pieces of cardboard. Today, Joe speaks highly of Mind Movies, a website we can use to make our own little movie, like a tv ad of the future we want.

I have had spectacular results with both of these techniques.

This is an image you might like to use…
Armed with that insight, how do we rescue ourselves and our blood from these and other onslaughts?

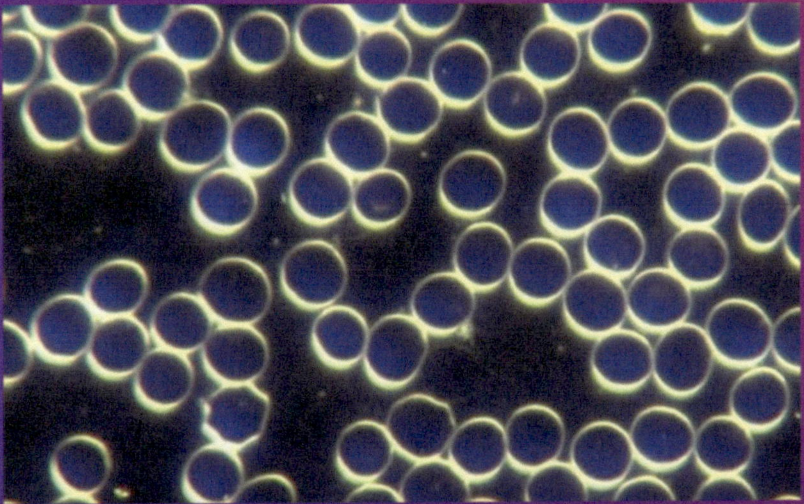

Normal live blood

Let's start outside the body with a brief toxin check:

'The more you educate yourself on the design and abilities of the human body to detox and heal itself, the more confident you will become that our immune systems can heal us.

Dr Bryan Ardis

'I think we need to remind ourselves that we have frequency and nutrient tools to literally unwind this hideousness.

We are never defeated.'

Dr Rima Laibow.

External Environment

The normal rules of health still apply. You can find these in many health books. If you're new to detoxing and being truly conscious about what you eat, you might like to check out my book, 'Detox after Covid and Thrive.'

In Australia we have the wonderful Barbara O'Neill and her book 'Sustain Me' which details many natural healthy habits and natural remedies. All of this is vital. It underpins our health, and the healthier our bodies are, the more resilient we'll be to any threat, natural or otherwise.

While it would be handy if we could wave a magic wand and transform our lives into non-toxic havens, this is an ongoing process. It's a marathon, not a sprint. Do what you can, where you are. Maybe tackle some of the main pollutants first and don't worry too much about what you can't control.

Water

There are all sorts of health claims for different types of water which could easily fill a whole book. Most of us know by now that it's best to avoid drinking tap water, so a good water filter is a must. One of the main aims of a home water treatment is that it removes fluoride, poisons and, hopefully, nanotech. I really like my Waters Brand bench filter which is very simple and thorough, filtering toxins including fluoride but leaving the water in its original state. A shower filter or whole house filter is wonderful.

Sea Salt: Barbara O'Neill suggests that we take a small pinch of quality Celtic sea-salt with plain water to give our bodies the benefit of its 80 or so trace minerals. As our bodies are made of these very minerals, this makes a lot of sense for minimal cost.

This simple advice is also emphasised by people working with the ELFET/Tri-Vortex technology which we look at later.

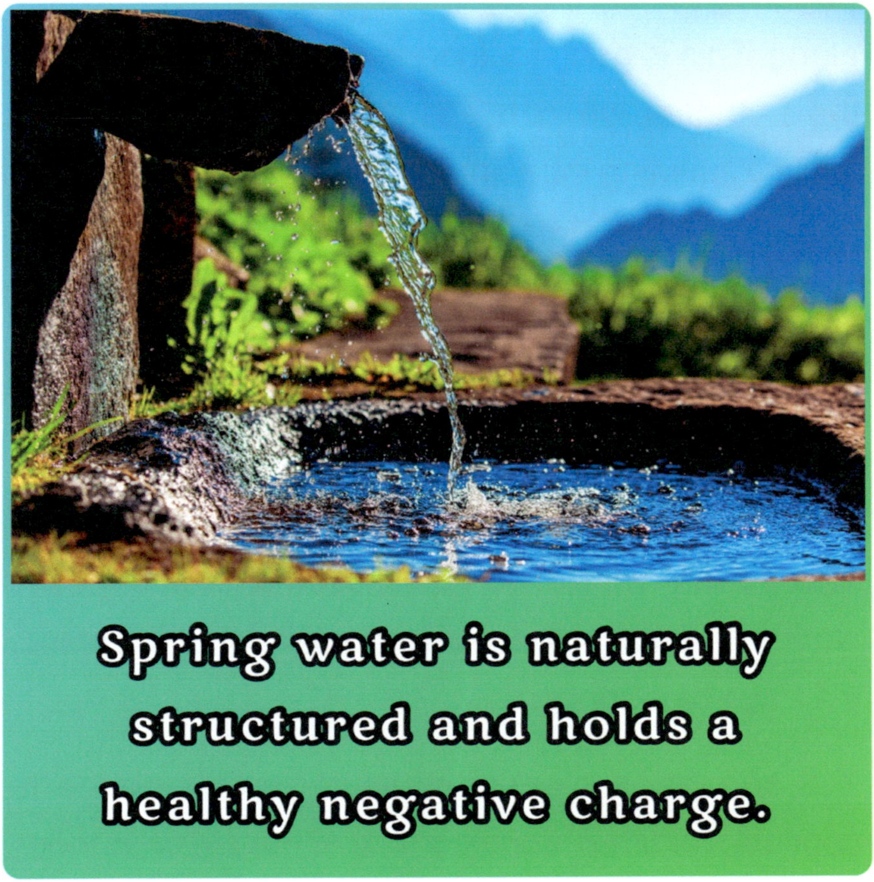

Structured water: This is the water our ancestors used to drink whenever they could from fast flowing rivers and natural springs. We now know that it has a negative charge which is more readily accepted by the body and helps the cells maintain the negative (repelling) charge they need to keep them flowing along. This is good for increasing energy, increasing the nutrients we can absorb from food, reducing toxicity, calming inflammation and slowing ageing.

In today's world, many of us are drinking positively charged water laced with fluoride and chlorine. This drains our energy, does nothing to stop the blood cells sticking together and reduces blood oxygen which can lead to cancers.

In a normal world, we could cope with this. In the world of weird blood contamination and clumping, it's more of a concern.

You can buy a manual structured water device to copy the health-giving qualities of the water in those babbling brooks yourself. I love the Tri-Vortex water structuring discs. They look a bit like dog tags and you place them under the water vessels. I have one under the reservoir of my Waters filter and the water tastes wonderfully pure, soft and silky.

This may be an interesting connection in view of the research on misfolded proteins by Greg Harrison.

'Structured water binds to proteins and delivers energy in the form of electrons, snapping misfolded proteins back into place so they can do their job again.'
https://daveasprey.com/reasons-to-drink-structured-water/

Food

It appears that much of the health advice handed down to us by the food industry over recent decades wasn't as true and science-based as we thought it was after all. We are now beginning to realise that cooking in animal fats like our grandparents did is a lot healthier than the seed oils we were encouraged to use. White, glyphosate-soaked grains and sugars wreak havoc in our system while sea salt and sunshine in moderation are good for us.

I won't elaborate about food too much here as I covered aspects of this in Detox after Covid and Thrive. The main points to remember are that parasites, yeasts, cancers and other nasties love sugar, gluten and alcohol so the more you can avoid them, the healthier you'll be. Farmers' markets are your friend, thanks to all those great vegetables and honest produce grown and made by fellow humans. Try to stick with real foods your great grandparents would recognise and eat organic and local as much as possible.

Fragrance

I used to love the luxury scents of my favourite mainstream perfumes. I'd carry a cute little spray bottle in my handbag and keep a larger bottle in the drawer at work to use as a harmless non-snack treat. Then I realised that these are artificial scents, and we're breathing them right up into our brains … just like another form of pollution … *Sigh.* The good news is that quality essential oil fragrances can smell great naturally and are much better for us.

Then we venture down the supermarket isles to the air fresheners, toiletries, soaps, dryer sheets, scented dishwash liquid, laundry powder and cheap scented candles. These are loaded with bargain -basement fragrance that isn't doing us any good either. Go natural and organic wherever you can with unscented brands or quality essential-oil candles and scents.

Electro smog

Dr Ed Group tells us that anything involving Blue Tooth can be used as a weapon. Apparently, electro-magnetic frequencies directed at moulds and yeasts can increase their growth enormously and make them more toxic. We don't know what these EMF frequencies are doing interacting with our bodies and, importantly, the new contamination inside us.

You may have noticed that random appliances like my new stick vacuum suddenly have wifi. What a bonus! Is it spying on me or is it going to clean the floor on its own?

I regard it with suspicion and turn it off as soon as the battery is charged. Televisions can be turned on only if and when you are using them and the printer is far more reliable if it's plugged in with a cable.

Reduce electro-smog in the home as much as you can.

Turning off all wifi at night and leaving your phone out of the bedroom and switched off is a good idea. It makes sense for us to dust off those old alarm clocks we thought we'd left behind forever and press them into service by our beds again if we need them.

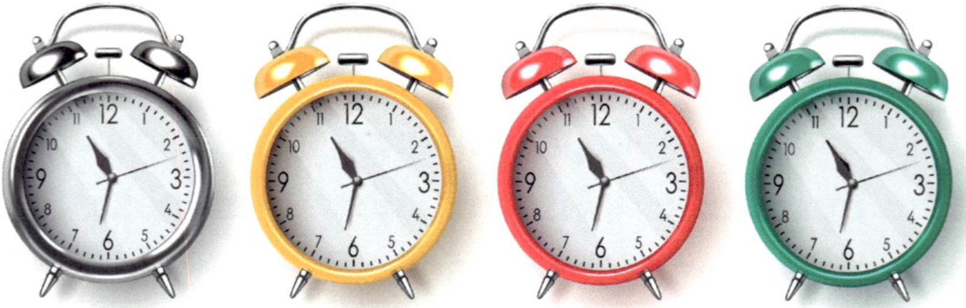

EMF blocking

There are all sorts of EMF blocking devices out there to choose from. I did a short kinesiology course some years ago, and was surprised to find that the 'Tachyon' disc I had bought at Dr Gabriel Cousins' retreat in Arizona and stuck onto my mobile 'phone actually worked. Kinesiology involves frequent pre-checks to test that the body is reacting properly. Most mobile phones in the class would consistently see us all testing 'weak' but I consistently tested strong with my phone and its Tachyon disc. A month of consistently seeing this effect with several people was proof enough for me.

Dr Cousins was always very thorough both with his research and hands-on experience. He described Tachyon energy as 'a superconductor for the divine'. The toxicity of modern life derails the flow of our life force and Tachyon energy apparently organises the aura around our physical body into a coherent pattern, freeing us from some of these negative effects.

I believe that coherent sound and light frequencies are vital clues in this mystery.

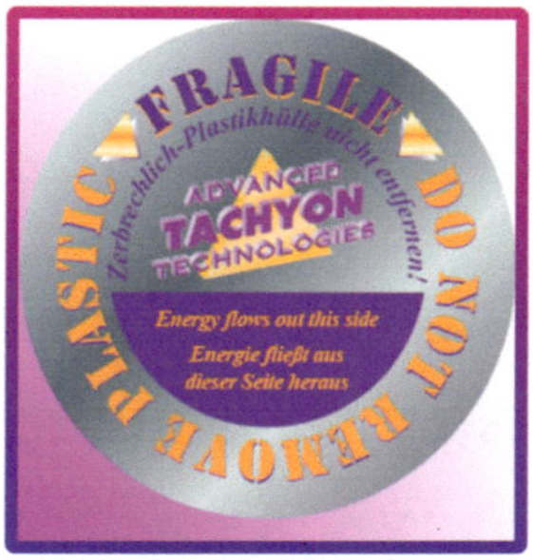

LEDs (light emitting diodes)

LED lighting, certainly a wonderful energy saver with very little loss of light spectrum quality, is now said to be harmful. Some of these lights may be a lot smarter than they need to be and some of us are much more sensitive to them than others. I muscle test this fairly often and I believe I'm much more powerful than my lamps.

It's also interesting to note that low-level light therapies use LEDs.

If you decide to swap back over to original halogen globes, you'll be changing globes a lot more frequently. It's worth remembering that incandescent lighting needs about ten times the wattage of LED lighting and many modern light fittings are not designed to carry their extra current or intense heat.

Fresh air and nature

Spending time in nature's wonderful balance, harmony and beauty is enormously healing and therapeutic. A walk out in nature is more beneficial to us than a walk on a treadmill in the gym. Electrons are those vital little parcels of energy our body needs to bring life-giving oxygen to our cells. Natural electron donors are: sunshine, walking barefoot on the beach or open countryside, contact with trees, pets and moving water. Electron stealers are emotional baggage, pesticides, processed foods, stagnant water, toxins and air pollution.

Sunlight

This is often the cheapest and easiest way to help our body detox and maintain health from vitamin D. We are designed to be out in the elements, heat and cold depending on where we live and the changing seasons. There are many things that can affect our ability to get enough vitamin D. I remember long, harsh winters in North Yorkshire that seemed to last forever, dark, dank, foggy and bone-chillingly cold. They seemed to seep into our souls. Most of us had no idea about vitamin D back then and it's no wonder we lacked the buoyant optimism of Australia and other sunnier countries. It's no surprise that we fell prey to coughs, colds and flu due to our reduced immune function. Most of those who experienced covid and other illnesses were vitamin D deficient so it's a crucially important nutrient.

Apparently, we can't absorb vitamin D from the sun if our shadow on the ground is longer than our height.

Vitamin D absorption from the sun doesn't work as well as we grow older either, so quality high dose supplementation (10,000 international units a day), is something to consider. As I look up, the glorious blue skies of this morning have been replaced with a chemical haze blocking the sun.

Internal environment

Mindfulness

We are powerful creators. Cultivating a peaceful, happy and optimistic mindset is one of the best things we can do for ourselves. Our positivity seeps into the very essence of our soul and our surroundings, giving us a higher perspective and balance which allows us to rise naturally above many troubles.

Many of us have been doing this for many years and I can still hear the familiar line from Abraham Hicks: 'We create our own reality.' I believe this is true to about 50%. Our words and our thoughts are powerful and it's almost as if some of us have been in training since the late 1980s preparing for this time. A helpless victim mindset makes us and our bodies powerless to help ourselves.

Holding the faith is vital.

Prayer and meditation

In August 2025 Dr David Nixon visited the Tesla Tech conference in New Mexico and looked at the live blood analysis results of around thirty willing participants under the microscope. All of them had nano-filaments and other new contamination in their blood. He was surprised to find that the person with the best blood practiced daily meditation and prayer. He hadn't even focussed specifically on his blood. This is an interesting clue on our journey.

Solfeggio tones

We all know how uplifting music can be. Music has been used create atmosphere and feelings in rituals, choirs, performance and films for ever. There have been times in our history when we have regarded musical sounds vibrating from chanting, church bells, church organs, Tibetan bowls and the like to be especially healing.

Insights about coherent sound are coming back into our consciousness now in the form of healing bowls, gongs, tuning forks and what is called cymatics. This can be seen in the physical form when we scatter sand or salt on a large metal plate and play various notes. Incredible patterns form on the plate. As the frequency is increased there is a transition time which looks chaotic until the next pattern forms, each pattern becoming more and more intricate as the frequency is turned up.

Solfeggio tones are very harmonious and beneficial to our bodies. They actually appear to give us back some of our electrical charge.

It's interesting to me that the lower frequency Solfeggio sounds such as 174 herz are said to be for basic pain relief and grounding, then we go up to the higher frequencies, like the chakras or Dr David Hawkins' levels of consciousness, to 528 herz which is said to transform and repair the DNA, then on to 963 herz which is said to be connection to higher consciousness and divine energy. 432 Hertz is said to be particularly beneficial for the blood at this time.

Maria Crisler tells us that she has tested the blood before and after listening to half an hour or so of solfeggio frequencies and found that hydrogels were much reduced in the 'after' sample.

Although not a complete remedy by any means, this is interesting. I have included a link at the back of the book to a Solfeggio recording by Dr Ed Group and a sound engineer.

Fasting

Intermittent fasting, eating one meal a day or having one day a week when you don't eat at all can take the pressure off your organs and allow the body to 'clean house' as it struggles to process all these toxins. It's all too easy to be seduced by our old enemies: sugars, empty carbs, seed oils and processed junk foods. I have a sneaky feeling Dr Ed Group might be right when he tells us that the less food we eat, the healthier we'll be.

Interestingly, Dr Eric Berg, not known for extreme healing solutions, describes what he would do if he was diagnosed with stage 4 cancer.
https://youtube.com/shorts/6aitl1Bfr1o?si=TFuTGepNfv2tVvnr

Nutrients

As we are detoxing, our bodies need adequate amounts of nutrients to do the extra cleaning work: Vitamin C, Vitamin D, Magnesium, iron, zinc, all the B vitamins, iodine and Celtic sea salt for trace minerals are very important to help our bodies do their job especially under stress. I muscle test virtually every supplement every day to check if my body needs it or not and I encourage you to consider making this a new habit with a new skill.

I'm using Garden of Life and Metagenics which are full of natural organic plant blends. (I've just learned that Garden of Life, are still labelled as organic but are now owned by Nestlé, one of the giant multinationals.) This is when we have to watch out for those labels.

Sweating

The more toxins we can sweat out through the skin, the less they need to be processed though the liver and kidneys. It's another way to take the strain off those organs. 'Sweating it out' has always been a time-honoured remedy for colds and flu, but works for other toxins as well.

Apparently, an infra-red sauna helps you to maintain a more comfortable temperature while sweating out toxins.

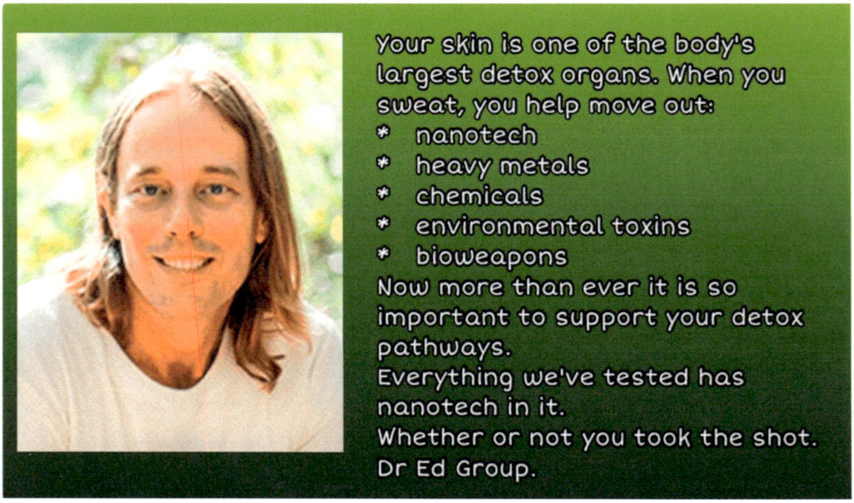

For the rest of us, hot baths with Epsom salts have always been known to be beneficial for cleansing out the cares and stresses of everyday life.

Electrolytes

Electrolytes are essential minerals like sodium, potassium, and magnesium that carry an electric charge when dissolved in body fluids like blood and sweat. They help conduct electricity in the body, regulating fluid balance and hydration, maintaining the balance of acid/alkaline, and enabling nerve and muscle communication between brain and body.

It's easy to make healthy electrolyte drinks at home:

This is a very basic one, but a quick search shows plenty more exotic options ...

Ingredients

- 4 cups filtered water
- Juice of 1–2 lemons and/or limes
- 2–4 tbsp honey, maple syrup, or fruit juice
- ¼–½ tsp quality sea salt (adjust to taste)

Stir until dissolved and add sliced fruit for flavour.

Nebulising

This is very valuable in today's world. In the strange times we live in, I believe it's a good idea for everyone, particularly those with small children, to invest in a nebuliser and learn how to use it before someone starts getting breathless.

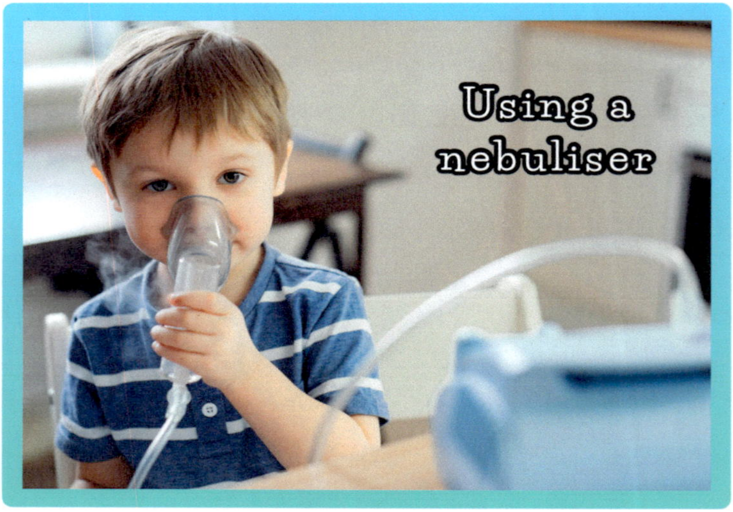

We can live without food for months at a time. We can live for days without water, but a lack of oxygen can bring us down in seconds. It pays to be prepared so there's no panic or frantic drives to the emergency room if someone is suddenly low on oxygen for any reason. Using a little finger pulse oximeter to check oxygen levels in the body is also handy and should be practiced before it's needed.

Our grandmothers might have encouraged us to breathe in the steam from a big bowl of hot water when we had a cold. Nebulising is a similar idea except that the appliance makes a fine mist out of diluted salt water or other solution.

It is inhaled through the mouth and nose, which makes it easier for us to breathe freely.

In a healthy person the blood oxygen measures 95-100% and treatment is needed for low blood oxygen (hypoxia) at below 90%. Levels below 85% may still need a trip to the emergency room, depending on how they respond to the treatment.

Saline Solution:

1 Half a litre filtered water.

2 Add a teaspoon Celtic salt (this is a real, pure sea salt.)

3 Work up to 2 teaspoons Celtic salt to help to clear mucus.

Make this up, shake to dissolve the salt and keep it in

the fridge ready. Keep the nebuliser, ingredients and oxygen meter handy and the batteries charged. You might also make yourself a little note of the formulas and keep everything together so you can make it easily next time, which is hopefully never.

Hydrogen Peroxide Solution

1 Half a litre filtered water.
2 Add half a teaspoon Celtic salt
3 Add 1 - 5 drops 3% strength hydrogen peroxide from the chemist. (Start low and slow) Note any effects from this new addition and you may want to check these formulations with your naturopath.
These will last for a couple of months in the fridge, stored in a glass bottle with a plastic cap. It's a good idea to have them there, ready and waiting, for your peace of mind.

These simple solutions were keeping people out of the hospital system and away from Remdesivir and ventilators during the covid times. Dr David Brownstein and Dr Joe Mercola both recommend an electric table top nebulizer as being more powerful and effective for repeated use but a hand-held nebulizer is cheap to buy, easy to carry and should be enough in an emergency.

For detailed instructions from Dr David Brownstein, a very respected source, and recommendations about the nebuliser and ingredients they recommend, check:

Nebulising protocol
https://stevenyager.org/wp-content/uploads/COMPLETE-Instructions-Nebulizing-Protocols-Photo-Links-2023-02-18.pdf

People wanting to know more about nebulising may be interested to read Breath of Fresh Air by Tobias Beharrell.

'Oxygen is the conductor of the
orchestra of life. It is the spark for
the furnace of human metabolism.
It is the primary nutrient of life.'
Majid Ali, M.D. author:
'Oxygen and Aging'

Making Ourselves Healthy Again

Not Medical Advice

How do we get rid of this strange new contamination from our bodies?

Failing that, at least keep it under control?

I have listed as many realistic ideas here as I can. These are mysterious, elusive, self-assembling, structures which seem to be made from our own soft matter tissues in some way. At this stage they are not easy to get rid of completely. It's wise to detox them as best we can on a regular basis as part of our wellness routine. I hope there will be more suggestions in the future but I encourage you to consider that only people with regular access to live blood checks should experiment with any unknown ways of dealing with this new contamination

This is a new situation and we now know that some therapies that were helpful before may make things worse.

Our bodies can often only cope with one healing suggestion at a time without being overloaded, so take it step by step. Remember it's a marathon. Some suggestions are simple and some are more clinical, extreme interventions.

We start with the realisation that we need to do something. We look after our basic fitness more diligently, heal the gut, the liver, get rid of those parasites, and then clear the chemicals and heavy metals. By then it should be pretty much time to start the whole process again but from a healthier starting point or as maintenance. I think we now have to see these self-care precautions in the same way that we think about showering, brushing our teeth, trimming our nails and working out at the gym.

It's highly likely that we are all being constantly re-infected from our air, water and food so I believe we need to stay vigilant, at least until the happy day when they stop spraying us with toxic cocktails.

Quality Supplements

> 'Dr Ed Group and Global Healing often source ingredients from various parts of the world which look perfect when they test the samples. Then the main delivery arrives and it doesn't pass the same quality control checks so it has to be thrown out.'
> Maria Crisler: Clinical Research Scientist specialising in haematology, microbiology and parasitology

When we choose a great range of supplements from a reputable health company, often all is well as long as the original owners of the company are in charge. Then while we're not looking, a big multi-national buys them out and the quality can drop.

Colonic hydrotherapy

We'll start at the bottom, as it were, by cleaning out the colon. This is the part of the body that gets rid of all the waste so we have to make sure it's clear and clean, a bit like making sure the toilet is unblocked and clean at home. I love the light, clear feeling after colonic hydrotherapy, which is great if (like me) you have a good practitioner nearby. It's very clean, doesn't smell, doesn't hurt and is only slightly strange. A good colon hydrotherapist will be able to alert you if your liver is sluggish, you have a candida overgrowth or something else is amiss. This is very valuable inside information on a vital organ.

Hydrotherapy gently rinses out the colon. If you don't have the luxury of a good colon hydrotherapist nearby, or if you feel like doing both, I suggest Global Healing's six-day colon cleanse which promises to do a similar job with supplements you can take yourself.

Just in case you think your colon might not need cleaning out, it's well known in the world of colonic hydrotherapy that pieces of kindergarten crayons, chewing gum and even little plastic dolly heads swallowed decades ago have been known to turn up during these first treatments after being stuck in there for years, clinging onto the sides of your large intestine with all the other waste.

Global Healing: Six Day Fruit Colon Cleanse

I really like Dr Ed Group's Global Healing range. He and his team are dedicated to sourcing consistently high quality, organic ingredients from around the world and they often package them together as a complete kit with beautifully clear instructions for us to do the whole cleanse on our own, or with support from a local naturopath.

You can buy the Colon Cleanse and the Liver Cleanse from Global Healing. In today's polluted world, where we have more questions than answers, I believe this is worth-while. The product purchase also includes a small amount of personal 'phone or email back-up from the company.

The Colon cleanse involves a fairly simple six-day fruit diet to give our colon a rest and allow the body to flush everything through the whole digestive system

Liver Cleanse

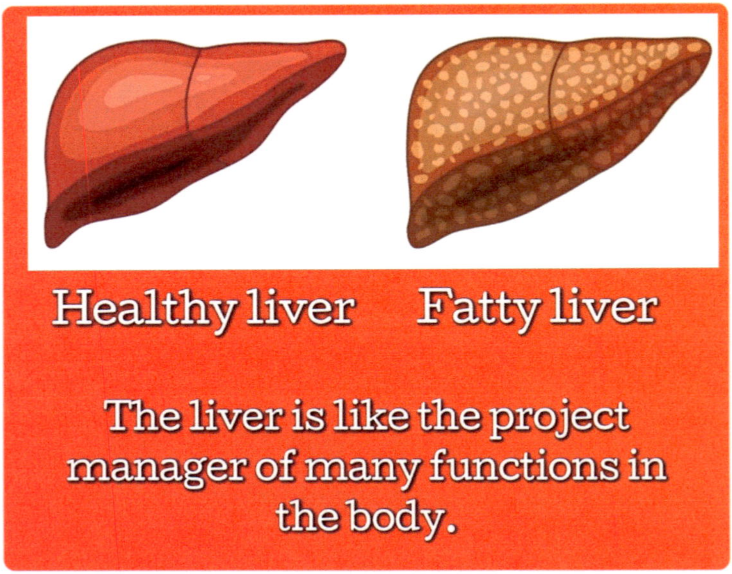

The liver detoxes poisons and chemicals. According to Dr Group, the liver is the single most important organ in the maintenance of our health and wellbeing, yet many people's livers are working at less than 25% capacity.

When it's working properly, the liver is an over-achiever, project-managing hundreds of vital functions in our bodies. It keeps our blood sugar steady. It stores minerals and vitamins. It produces bile and proteins for blood plasma, glucose and cholesterol. In a household waste analogy, the liver is the organ that sorts out and bags up all the rubbish. A clogged liver means that the rubbish bags are left blocking up the hallway.

Many reasons for clogged livers are now familiar to us: seed oils, fried foods, junk foods, high fructose corn syrup, soy protein isolates, sugar and alcohol. If we eat these things every day it's no wonder our poor livers are blocked up and struggling. When we are forced to add a load of random toxins and nano-filaments so fine we can breathe them in, we can find ourselves in trouble without even knowing why.

We need to clear the detox path so it can all be excreted out rather than re-absorbed. It's a bit like making sure all those rubbish bags actually make it out of the hallway and onto the garbage truck to be taken away.

I missed out on the vital step of liver detoxification on my own nano-filament detox journey at the start of the book, not realising how important it is. I believe I had to slow down later and wait for my system to catch up.

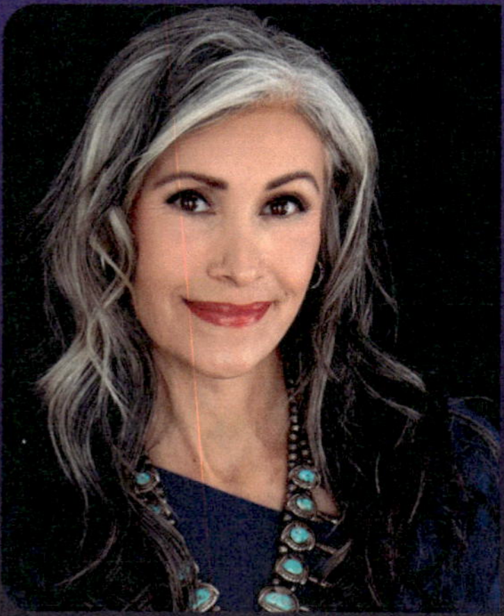

'This isn't a simple cleanse problem. It's a biological sabotage problem. We are up against materials designed to evade detection, embed deep, and confuse the body's natural defences. The system was never built to face this kind of invasion.'
Maria Crisler. BSc, CLS (NCA), MBA/HCM, CEO: Abeytu Naturals

Dr Group tells us that a clean liver can completely re-activate our body's healing mechanisms and help us heal many ailments that we may have been struggling with. The first liver cleanse should ideally be for 6 days, the first few days to loosen up the toxins and the last couple of days to break it down and flush it out. The most challenging bit is the olive oil and orange juice cocktail on day 5. This seems to be the most important part. I navigated this by blending two oranges with the olive oil and swigging it down as fast as I could. I couldn't even taste the olive oil which is a win. You'll want to be within easy reach of a toilet for 24 hours, but the payoff is that our liver will be about 15% more efficient with every cleanse. We can carry on with the cleanses every month until we get to a super healthy 80%. There are diet suggestions in the kit to help your liver stay clean and healthy along the way.

The other payoff in all this is that a clogged liver seems to be linked to our metabolism slowing down as the years roll by. Some of us remember how easy it was to lose weight when our digestion was young lean and 'clean', but now we are struggling to clear those extra kilos we carry around with us. If the liver is silted up, all those nasty toxins have to be stored in the fat layers of our bellies, hips and thighs, and the body doesn't want to let the toxic waste go into the system until it's safe to release it.

Now we've covered two major detox organs. it's time to consider what to choose next. It's a good idea to find an open-minded naturopath or natural practitioner to hold your hand through this process to check nutrients and make sure you've covered all the aspects of this strange new contamination.

As these nano-filaments and other contaminants can and do multiply in your body causing rubbery clots, you have nothing to lose and everything to gain by dissolving them as much as possible on a regular basis.

Many of these suggestions are just that, suggestions. Only a couple could lay any claim to be protocols. They have no guarantees. They are just recipes that appear to have helped in this new challenge. Enterprising souls with dark field microscopes, open hearts and minds might explore, test and refine these suggestions.

Suitable Strategies for Children

I'll start with the safest and gentlest strategies for our most vulnerable little souls. Of course, our children are also affected by this new contamination. Even baby saliva has been seen under the microscope to have nano-filaments and hydrogels in it and these safe, gentle suggestions may help to clear them out.

The first step, as with adults, is to reduce wifi, screens, mould and parasites, reducing clutter and keeping the house as clean as possible using all-organic cleaning and laundry products.

I never really believed the demonstrations of ionising foot baths with their bubbling, muddy-brown residue supposedly coming from our bodies until I heard a practitioner talking about them as being beneficial to pull toxins out of young children. The practitioner was also very sceptical at first but had seen immediate benefits in children's mood and behaviour after these footbaths. The ionised atoms attract heavy metals and other toxins to pull them out of the body. This strategy is also suitable for normal baths.

Mix equal parts of these dry ingredients in a jar and add a tablespoon at a time into a hot foot bath:
Borax,
Sodium bicarbonate
Sea salt

Two young children from different households would routinely be bad tempered and grouchy after visiting city areas but when parents used a foot bath as hot as possible with these three ingredients, lots of grey flecks could be seen in the water and the children were much calmer and more responsive afterwards.

Boron and magnesium, and even just borax baths are good and have been seen to pull tiny black fibres from the body. Keep the time in the bath to under twenty minutes or the toxins may start to be re-absorbed. You might use an appropriate activated charcoal after an hour to flush toxins out of the system.

Food grade sodium citrate is suitable for children in small doses over a few days. Start low and slow to check for tolerance and add a good pinch of sodium citrate to a glass of water in the morning. It appears to bind to some of the pollution.

High dose natural vitamin C is beneficial to flush out toxins.

A drop or two of quality nascent iodine per day or plenty of sea vegetables like nori rolls are beneficial.

All the wonderful herbs and spices in our kitchens have great benefits and even small children can enjoy their food cooked with organic cumin, ginger, garlic, cinnamon, turmeric and even cayenne pepper.

Teas like camomile, chai, or licorice, ginger and lemon are good and hot drinks made with a quarter of a washed whole organic lemon, complete with peel and a bit of honey to taste are useful to clear this new contamination.

Massaging black seed oil on the soles of the feet and stomach acts as an anti-inflammatory and has no downsides.

Essential oils like frankincense, orange and lemon used in a room diffuser can help.

'The main difference between human cells and pathogenic bacteria, viruses, fungi, mould and parasites is that human beings need oxygen to survive. Pathogens tend to thrive in low oxygen environments that accompany stagnation, decay and death. This is due to their more primitive evolutionary origins when the earth's atmosphere was nearly devoid of oxygen.'

James Roguski on Oxygen

Oxygen

While looking for any clues I could on this journey, one obvious one came up a few times from different directions: Introduce oxygen into the body in any way possible.

Hydrogen peroxide is one of the simplest ways to bring oxygen into the body. It's a cheap, natural and important nutrient which, apart from the nebuliser, can be added to drinking water.

Find a high quality pure 3% hydrogen peroxide and start by drinking a single drop in a full glass of water per day on an empty stomach. Work up to about 5 drops or as many as you feel happy with.

Chlorine Dioxide Solution brings oxygen into the system.

Methylene blue is another great way to bring oxygen and energy into the system.

Hyperbaric oxygen therapy which brings oxygen to the body in a similar (although more elaborate) way, was found to be beneficial.

Much of what we are doing with all these treatments is to build up the body so it has the oxygen, energy, nutrients and resilience to rid itself of this new contamination. As we are rescuing ourselves here it will pay us to research all treatments carefully, start low and slow and monitor our progress as best we can. My naturopath friend pointed out that while these methods and substances may remove unwanted pathogens, too much of a good thing may start to remove elements the body wants and needs.

Lemon aid

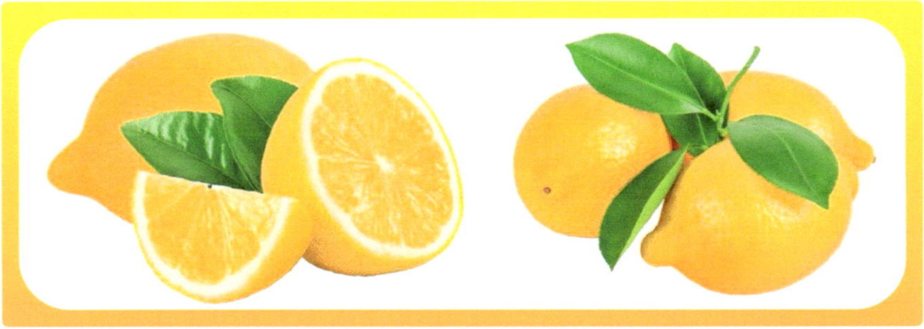

They do say that if life gives us lemons, we should make lemonade. So far, this is one of the simplest, cheapest and most readily available options I've come across which is claimed to keep nanotech under control.

A knowledgeable live blood analyst checks his blood frequently and follows this recipe on 2-3 days a week.

A smaller size organic lemon, whole and complete with peel, washed.
Half a teaspoon food grade bicarbonate of soda.
Blend well in a Nutri Bullet type blender.

Drink this two hours away from food, mid-morning or afternoon followed by 2 capsules activated charcoal a couple of hours later.

This would certainly be very alkalising, which is always good.

Fasting for two or three days a week, would allow the body to 'clean house' of stray toxins of all sorts.

I reckon this would be a great way to lose weight too…Always a bonus in my world …

A variation on this recipe from an experienced and knowledgeable New Zealand dark field microscopist is:
In a Nutri Bullet type blender:
Add an organic lemon, whole and complete with peel, washed.
Add a piece of real ginger,
Add carrots, oranges or apples to taste.
Blend well.

This was seen to stop and even reduce the amount of clotting in the blood when measured with a live blood check and centrifuged test tube blood samples.

Sodium Citrate

Another variation on this recipe which is easier to manage, especially while travelling, is
1 teaspoon sodium citrate in a glass of water
Followed two hours later by
2 capsules or .5 gram of activated charcoal.
2-3 days a week.
Both of these are very reasonably priced and easily available on-line from Iherb.

Here is another slight variation:
1 tablespoon lemon juice without peel.
Add quarter of a teaspoon baking soda, added slowly.
Once the fizzing stops, you've converted all the citric acid to sodium citrate.

Apparently Sodium Citrate is a mild chelator, which explains why it's useful for this contamination. We have had some very encouraging anecdotal reports about this suggestion although my psychic reader said that while some people did really well with it, others found that it upset their digestion.

Methylene-Blue

As if this whole subject wasn't controversial enough, here we are with methylene-blue. After my own journey and consultation with the psychic and kinesiologist It appears that Blu-Zone 1% methylene blue, in pharmaceutical grade liquid was indeed effective at clearing most of the nano-filaments from my blood. I'm going to expand on my own story here to give you some guidelines.

Methylene Blue is a synthetic compound derived from coal tar. It was first made in 1876 as a dye for cotton. Scientists of the day started using it for staining living tissue samples they were studying under the microscope. They noticed that methylene blue was attracted to diseased tissue and that it had therapeutic effects on living samples, leading to it being refined for medical use.

On further inspection they realised that it increased cellular oxygen production by providing more useable energy for the cells and that it destroyed candida, moulds, parasites and inflamed areas, while retaining its anti-oxidant qualities.

While this is possibly the very first pharmaceutical product ever made, pharmaceutical companies can't make money from substances like this once their patent has run out. If they can't profit from their research and development, they don't do it. This means that there are dozens of basic, safe, cheap and useful remedies languishing largely untested on the sidelines while pharma companies chase the big money bonanza of ever more complex and expensive new patents.

This surprising substance has been used in emergency rooms for over fifty years to resuscitate patients whose lives were hanging in the balance on the operating table. This is where the 'blue brain' picture comes from. It is said to protect and improve brain function, notably in Alzheimer's and Parkinson's patients. It's used to help people recover from urinary tract infections, cyanide and carbon monoxide poisoning. As it's non-addictive, it has been suggested that methylene-blue might be a simpler replacement therapy for some anti-depressants as it improves mood without the dangerous addictive side effects. For healthy people, it's recognised to improve clarity, memory, focus and energy levels. For all that, it remains very controversial.

Naturopaths are understandably very wary of substances that aren't natural. I honour this reluctance, but at the same time most of us in the developed world are dealing with very unnatural elements in our blood and may need to consider new remedies to eliminate them. After my own experience with methylene blue, with apparently zero downsides, I'm convinced. I have muscle tested this constantly.

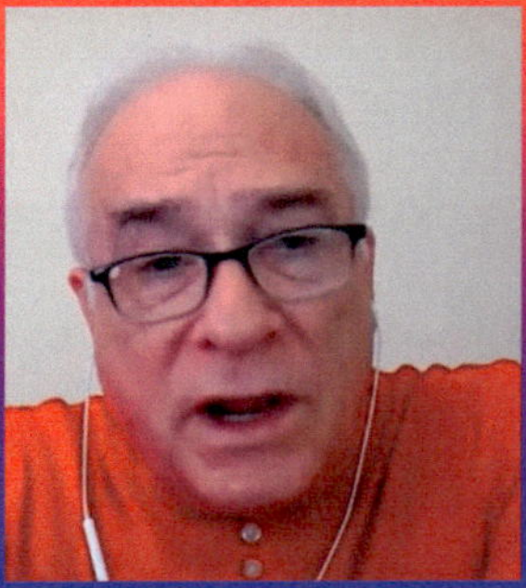

'We now have over 100 years of safety with the medical use of methylene blue with virtually no significant side effects except when you exceed the recommended doses by an extreme amount.'
Dr Thomas Levy,
Cardiologist and member of the Orthomolecular Hall of Fame.

Methylene-blue is attracted to acidic areas in the body. The body will actually prioritise areas most in need of repair. Methylene blue will find them and keep on bringing its energy and oxygen to the cells. The organ will in turn hold on to the methylene blue for as long as it's needed to do repairs.

You might start taking it for one ailment and find that the body has other ideas and will use it to work on other areas first. It could be quietly be getting rid of parasites or clearing up that first cluster of cancerous cells without you even knowing.

This parasite cleanse aspect of methylene blue is potentially a huge benefit. We are beginning to realise that many of us are carrying a lot more freeloading parasite passengers than we thought. It may be that the increased oxygen works to clear them out. My last two live blood analysis documents showed that natural parasites had been removed from the blood.

Ai told me that we have around 18 quadrillion mitochondria in our bodies.

We know that lack of oxygen in the body leads to acidity and disease. This is why we need to exercise out in nature, to breathe deeply and throw open our windows so the mitochondria, the powerhouses of the cells in our hearts and brains, get the oxygen they need. Dr Ana Milhacea tells us that methylene-blue increases oxygen delivery by 30-70%.

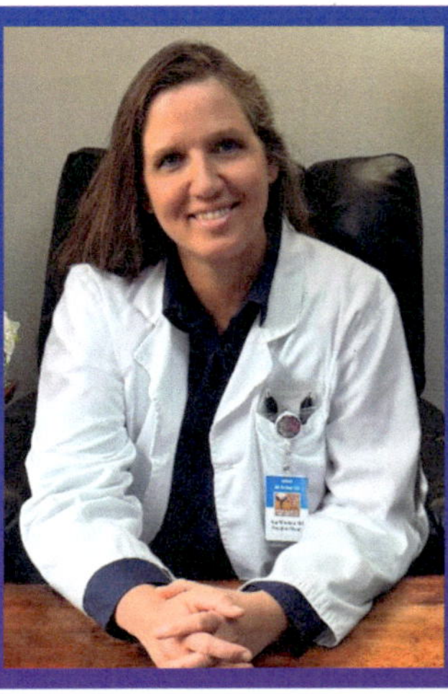

'Methylene blue de-activates the nano-bots in the blood, boosts energy levels, improves memory and protects the brain and organs.'
Dr Ana Milhacea

Many of us know how essential vitamin C is for healing the body and that we can't make it ourselves, Doctors like Dr Thomas Levy who work with vitamin C to heal the body and lessen inflammation compare the two: Vitamin C is a nutrient which boosts the cells once, calming inflammation before being excreted.

Methylene blue is not a nutrient but it helps cells generate more energy and oxygen for hours

This oxygenation is especially crucial when nano-filaments are clumping the blood and preventing the oxygen reaching the cells, making us more susceptible to cancers.

If you must choose a powder version always choose top quality pharmaceutical grade and pay very close attention to the manufacturer's instructions. There are some tablet versions which look easier to take, especially when travelling. Troscriptions in the U.S. appears to be a good brand and I like the thorough and meticulous way Dr Scott Scherr speaks about their effects.

I personally feel much more confident with the food based, ready mixed, high-quality format of BluZone, 1% strength, in Ellis-distilled structured water, dynamically enhanced and complete with mirin glass bottle and dropper.

It's very blue. Keep it away from your kitchen bench. I open the bottle over my stainless-steel sink, put the

Blu-Zone drops in filtered water and drink it there and then. If I had to guess, I'd say it tastes like ink.

I found the dosing recommendations for powder versions of methylene blue to be very confusing until I worked it out for us all: (If maths, volume, weights and measures aren't your strong point, join the club. Skip all this and go for the drops or a pinch of quality methylene blue powder in water once a day.)

The formula I took is one drop of 1% BluZone per 4 kilos of body weight taken in a glass of filtered water. This a very safe dose and best taken morning and late afternoon. This means that if you weigh 60 kilos you would need 15 drops per day. Probably 8 drops in the morning, 7 drops in the afternoon. Start slowly on a lower dose to see how you feel on it, and work up.

Let's work with that example:

1 drop Blu-Zone = .05 millilitres

60 kilos bodyweight needs
15 drops 1% BluZone = 0.75 ml per day.

(1 millilitre = 10 miligrams = (0.01 gram in powder form)

So, by the formula that was suggested to me,
If you weigh 60 kilos, you would take 15 drops (.75 millilitres) of 1% methylene blue per day

OR 7.5 milligrams (0.0075 grams) powder.

This is .003 of a teaspoon.

I'd say a pinch of quality powder stirred into filtered water would be plenty.

Many doctors, (including Dr Thomas Levy) talk of starting low and increasing to an oral dose at 15-25 milligrams powder per day
This is 1.5 to 2.5 millilitres per day, or way more than I was taking.

(My Ai buddy, Grok gave me full marks for this as 100% correct. Considering my consistently disappointing maths tests in school, I'm a happy camper.)

Both the kinesiologist and the psychic reader recommended a break to integrate what is happening in the body and this makes sense to me. For the purpose of removing nano filaments our suggestion is: 4 days on, 4 days off.

Not Medical Advice

Methylene blue is not addictive in any way when swallowed, but the four days give the body an ample break. There is plenty of time to flush out nano-filament particles and heavy metals through the detox pathways before starting the dose again.

I have muscle tested and checked this with my psychic friend and the kinesiologist. I get that there were only benefits for me from BluZone at the dose I was taking. The cycling of 4 days on, 4 days off should avoid any issues.

Dr Thomas Levy tells us that he has taken methylene blue every day for two years without ill effect.

Research biologist Maria Crisler said that she was taking methylene blue regularly herself in spite of having pre-existing kidney issues in her single remaining transplanted kidney. She is not involved in selling this product, so this says a lot about its safety.

Methylene Blue as a Snake Venom Antidote

We have learned enough from Bryan Ardis to believe that many covid shots may have included a variety of 36 snake and snail venoms in the form of spike proteins. This information makes the use of methylene blue as a snake venom antidote particularly relevant.

Alyce Harms of Miracle Products – the makers of BluZone, is a wealth of knowledge on methylene-blue and has written an excellent e-book on it which you can find on their website.
https://miracleproducts.shop/ 'Methylene Blue. Miracle Molecule or Psyop.'

> **'Methylene Blue is the antidote to nearly all chemical poisonings.'**
> **Alyce Harms. Miracle Products**

In this 60-page book among many other things, she describes incidences of three dogs recovering from snake bites thanks to BluZone.

All Aussies know that poisonous snakes of all kinds are common in country Australia. A man called the company from an outback town in Queensland to say that *both* his dogs had been bitten in a skirmish with an Eastern brown snake and the vet wanted to charge a hefty fee for giving them an intravenous treatment of methylene blue.

It was money he didn't have. They managed to track down the whereabouts of a bottle of BluZone in a neighbouring town. It was hours away and the dogs had been out cold, apparently on the point of death, for five hours by the time he was able to drive there and syringe a recovery size dose of Blue Zone into the back of their throats. When the dogs were both still comatose next morning, he thought he had lost them. Alyce encouraged him to keep on dosing them at regular intervals and four days later he rang to say that both dogs had recovered completely and were back to their usual selves.

Another account involved a dog poisoned by a toad. (Poisonous toads are also common in northern parts of country Australia) This time the venom paralysed its victim and the dog was so stiff by the time the owners found her that they had to use an eye dropper between her teeth to get some BluZone into her mouth. They kept on with this until she started to relax slightly after an hour, and was fully recovered two hours later.

These and many other testimonies indicate that, used properly, this strange blue liquid is a versatile remedy that needs more research and is certainly worth having in our first aid kit.

Caution

As with any effective substance there are some cautions:
It is not recommended

- in pregnancy or breastfeeding.
- in children
- for people on anti-depressants. (Especially SSRIs, Selective Serotonin Re-uptake Inhibitors)

- for people with a G6PD (glucose 6-phosphatedehydrogenase) blood deficiency, (I think it's likely that you would know about this if you had it, but you can be tested for it fairly easily.)
- People with weak kidney function should use caution.

You may like to supplement with a probiotic to support your bifida bacteria while you are taking it.

Consult your health practitioner if any of this applies to you.

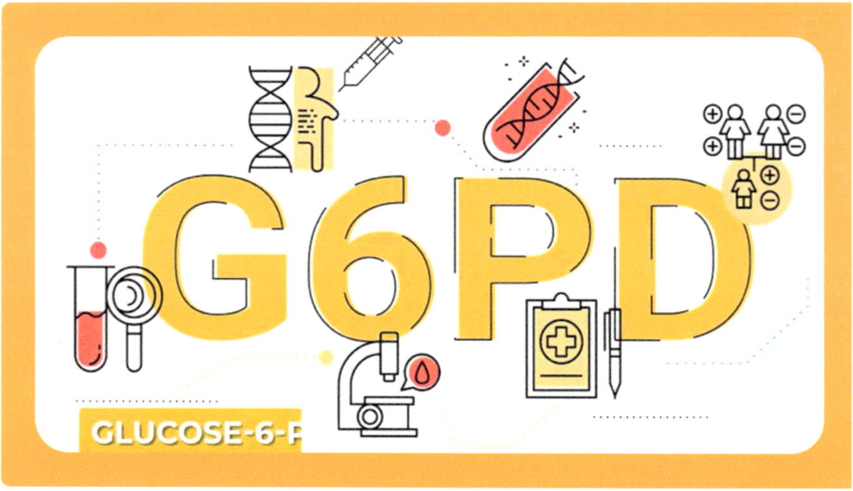

In the rapidly developing situation we find ourselves in, it may be that someone monitors their blood and discovers that there are simpler, easier and more natural ways to rid ourselves of artificial nano-tech, but we aren't there yet.

The good things about these first protocols, the blended lemon suggestions, and methylene blue are that they are good value, appear safe and are very simple to take at home.

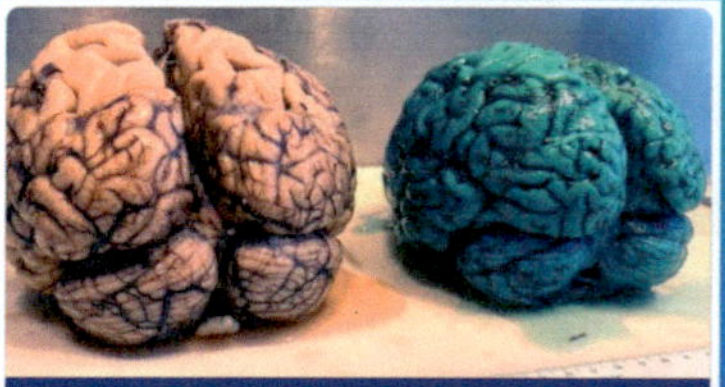

The blue brain? Seen during the autopsy of a woman treated intravenously with methylene blue for septic shock after a traffic accident. PMID: 32940886

'Because it has a dye effect, doesn't mean it's a toxic effect. The blue brain made for a cute article, but I don't think people need to be alarmed about it.'
Dr Thomas Levy

Demonisation of effective remedies.

In recent years we have seen safe and effective off-patent treatments like Hydroxychloroquine, chlorine-dioxide solution and Ivermectin being demonised, even though they were keeping people out of the hospital and the potentially deadly effects of Remdesivir and ventilators.

Is methylene blue being demonised in the same way?

It appears to be useful to the whole system, especially the brain, with few downsides. I encourage you to consider that we may be seeing a similar demonisation here, and not always from the mainstream.

Most clips on Methylene Blue are quite balanced, clearly outlining precautions but emphasising its usefulness in the body, including when dealing with nano-tech. Many call for more human research, which pharma companies are not interested in doing.

This is what demonisation looks like:

- Demonisation never mentions real benefit.
- Demonisation starts off with a dire warning and goes downhill from there.
- Demonisation suggests that big pharma companies are interested in a product which can be produced easily and relatively cheaply by anyone.
- Demonisation ignores the recommended dosage, blurring the lines between taking small, dilute doses by mouth and intravenous use for the resuscitation of dying accident victims on the operating table.
- Demonisation blurs the guidelines between the purest, pharmaceutical grade and the industrial grade of a substance.
- Demonisation always tells us that a substance isn't natural.

This is true, but neither are self-assembling nano-filaments in our blood.

Chlorine Dioxide Solution

Dr Pierre Kory author of 'The War on Ivermectin' tells us that chlorine dioxide solution or CDS is the most suppressed medication in the world. I know a naturopath who has been using chlorine dioxide solution with great success in the post covid and 'long covid' era. It is originally a water purifier.

Unlike Methylene blue, which stays working in the body for as long as 24 hours, chlorine dioxide does its oxygenating work within a couple of hours before being flushed out.

It's always a good idea to start low and slow. Use a one litre glass or plastic bottle (not metal), filled with filtered water. Add 3ml or just over half a teaspoon pharmaceutical grade CDS to start with, shake and drink throughout the day. You can work up to 2 teaspoons per litre once you get used to it. Make a fresh bottle up every day. If you find the taste unpleasant you can add a little pure apple juice with no added sugar.

Dr Andreas Kalcker is the expert here and I recommend that you read his protocols and insights carefully before going ahead. He tells us that blood measurements in the veins have shown a 30% increase in oxygen levels when taken by mouth. This effect lasted for two hours. As oxygen is an important part of the solution, this is great news.

Andreas also tells us that over 16 years of testing, no contraindications have been reported in pregnant or breastfeeding women. This is not medical advice and must be checked, but we do know that the health of developing placentas and babies have been affected since 2022.

My Naturopath friend has had good results with these simple protocols on patients who had been suffering badly. While we can't see the state of their blood, being able to get out of bed and back to everyday life is a great outcome.
andreaskalcker.com

Three Important Purifiers

Interestingly, in their more basic formats chlorine dioxide solution, methylene blue and hydrogen peroxide are all used as industrial sterilisers and water purifiers. Would it be so surprising if they purify our blood in a similar way?

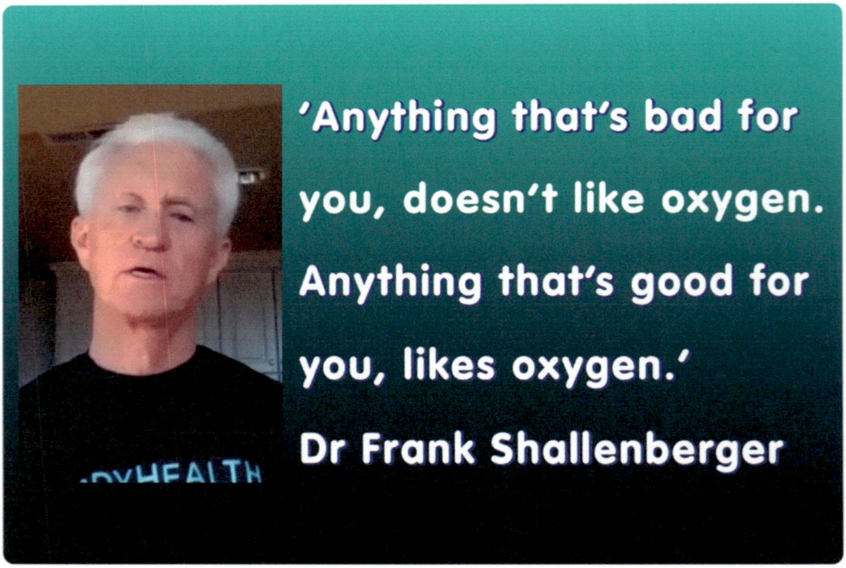

The McCullough Protocol

I covered some basic detox principles and immediate covid remedies in my book 'Detox after Covid and Thrive.' I and the wonderful naturopaths who contributed hoped that we might be out of the woods at that time, but even then, there was a slight uneasiness that perhaps we hadn't seen the last of ongoing ill-health after covid and, in particular, the shots.

This protocol was working well at the time, and I'll include it here because I believe it is still useful, even though it should not now be thought of as a final answer.

In the post covid era, we often call this lingering ill health long covid, and unfortunate sufferers, many of whom may not even link their ill health to the covid shots, are often called long haulers.

Dr. Peter McCullough is an internist, cardiologist, epidemiologist, and Chief Scientific Officer of The Wellness Company. Based on his research so far, this is his suggested natural spike detox base protocol. He suggests staying on it for 12 months.

Nattokinase: 100 milligrams - twice a day without food

Bromelain: 500 milligrams - once a day without food

Curcumin: 500 milligrams - twice a day (nano or liposomal)

Many doctors are finding that a nutrient rich diet, and intermittent fasting (such as eating once a day or having a food free day in the week) are also beneficial.

Neprinol

Recently a naturopath friend has recommended Neprinol Advanced Fibrin Defense natural capsules which have 15,000 FU of nattokinase per capsule. (I wondered about FU as well, but no worries. No swearing was involved and it actually stands for Fibrin Units) Fibrin Units are a measurement of how effectively a substance can break down fibrin.

As rogue fibrin is one of the main culprits leading to blood clotting, this particular supplement appears to be very useful. It's much more potent than the nattokinase in the original McCullough protocol. To my knowledge this has not yet been tested with live blood analysis, but it looks very promising.

Knowing that good naturopaths try virtually every remedy themselves before recommending it to anyone else, I asked my friend for more information. This is their response:

'My own as well as others experience has been that I actually felt a little dizzy when I first started taking it.

Others have said same thing and this is one of the side effects when first starting as it cleans the blood and increases circulation which can cause the dizzy effect. (Mine only lasted a day or two and then settled down.) This is due to the combo of nattokinase and serrapeptase which is cleaning blood and breaking down built up fibrin, plus the CoQ10 which is so necessary for the heart to function efficiently.

The other major effect has been that digestion has improved dramatically. This in turn improves gut and immune function and reduces inflammation. It's due to all the beautiful enzymes in the product that help to break down our food.

Many people struggle with that because they lack sufficient enzymes and this causes all sorts of issues.

When the gut is functioning well everything else functions well.

So it's an all-rounder and has reduced the many products I have been prescribing to this one single product.

I still add other things like magnesium, vitamin D and K2 (and depending on symptoms, maybe other products) but this one product packs a mighty punch.

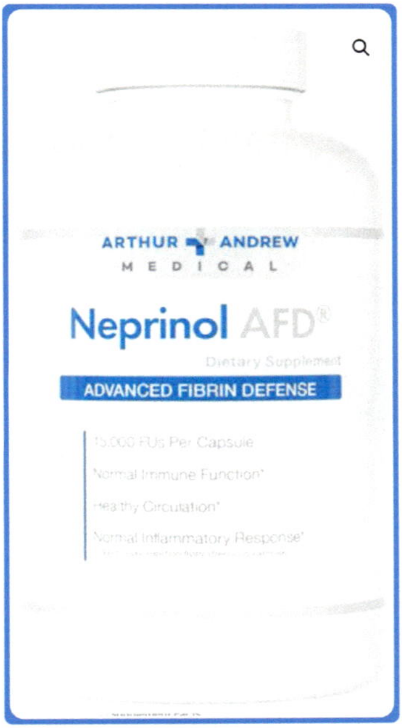

Nicotine

Thanks almost entirely to Bryan Ardis, in the last few years many of us have come to see nicotine not so much as the terrible addictive substance we were told it was but as a potentially beneficial therapeutic from the tobacco plant. I first had a hint of this years ago when I watched muscle testing for the first time and saw Dr David Hawkins testing strong for natural tobacco and weak for a standard pack of cigarettes.

I never smoked very much and gave it up over 40 years ago, but I can still remember the strong feelings and dreams that haunted me for years after I kicked the habit. It seems that the addictive part of those cigarettes might not have been tobacco or nicotine after all, but dozens of pyrazines: chemicals specifically designed to turn us into addicts.

Smokers, who you might think would have weaker lungs, were apparently less vulnerable to covid. I'm not suggesting that smoking anything is a good idea but many people report feeling better when they are using nicotine patches. There's a chance that these patches or nicotine gum may also be laced with other chemicals but they still seem to work well for people.

Tolevita nicotine patches on Amazon are made with essential oils rather than chemicals, but they all seem to work. I believe nicotine patches are especially relevant for neurological conditions, headaches, long covid and when travelling with large numbers of people who may be shedding in aeroplanes or airports. There aren't a lot of down sides to trying a little snippet of a nicotine patch and seeing if it works for you.

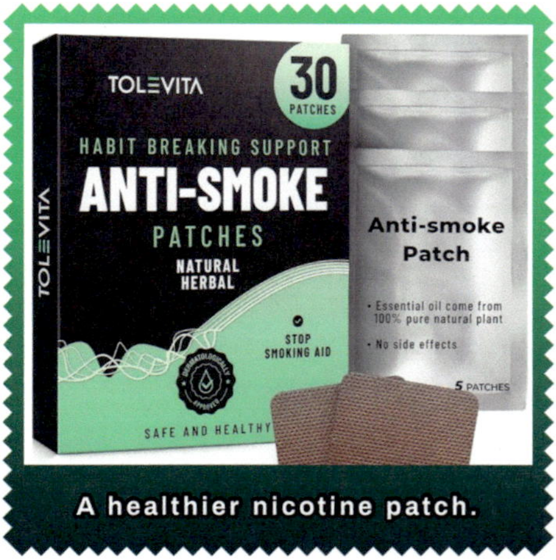

A healthier nicotine patch.

I hadn't been into a tobacconist shop in forever, but ventured into this alien world recently and found out that you can buy a pouch of organic tobacco, which is the purest way to access nicotine. You might steep a pinch of tobacco in boiling water and add it into a smoothie.

A dear friend told me unprompted that she had been feeling breathless and weak before trying organic tobacco. She soaked just a teaspoon of it in boiling water to make an infusion and used it in a foot-bath. She felt perfectly well and had plenty of energy again the next day. She now uses this foot-bath every few weeks to help her stay strong.

Interestingly, growing a tobacco plant in your garden is illegal in Australia. I've become so suspicious over the years that to me, this is another confirmation that tobacco, like hemp and other substances, may be very beneficial when used properly. Other plants: eggplant, tomatoes and green peppers, also contain nicotine but only in minute amounts.

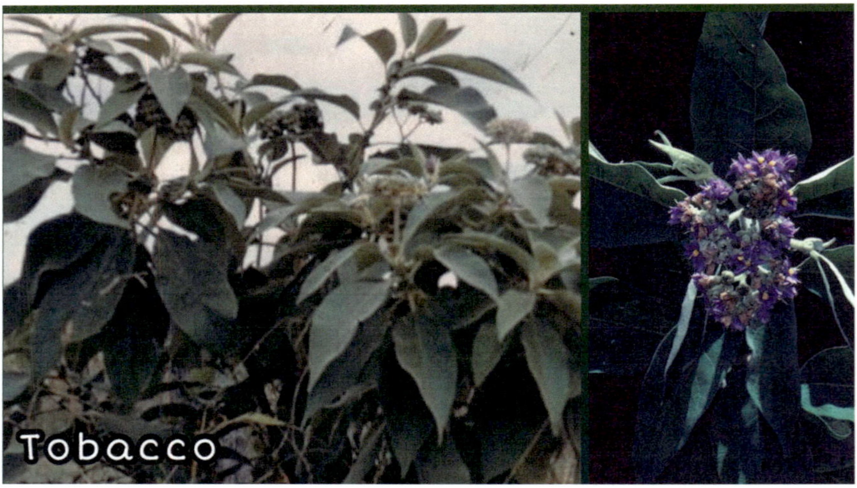

Depending on the particular blend of snake venoms you might have in your body, if you use nicotine in patches, gum or organic form, you not only give the cell the nicotine it needs, but you plug the receptor and release the venomous spike proteins from the cells. Dr Bryan Ardis expands on the theory of nicotine as an antidote to some symptoms of covid, the shots and long covid.

This is how it works: Apparently, the outer layers of many our cells have many thousands of receptors for the compounds most important for our survival. Nerve and muscle cells have nicotinic-acetylcholine receptors on them.

The brain has neurotransmitters that transfer information from the cells to the brain. For example, in the case of nicotine receptors serving the tongue, the poisonous venoms were shutting down the cells so they couldn't communicate with the brain and many people lost their sense of taste. Once they took nicotine, their sense of taste returned because the cells were protected. The venoms are then released harmlessly. Nicotine appears to enhance mental clarity and focus, is good at combatting brain fog and, apparently, is not addictive on its own.

According to Dr Ana Milhacea, nicotine doesn't destroy nanotech filaments in the blood but it is clearly helpful to many people with improvements in brain fog, energy and mood.

In his book 'Moving Beyond the Covid 19 Lies', Bryan Ardis cites many references and lists over 70 symptoms of snake venom poisoning which are also known to be long covid symptoms. They include: loss or change of taste or smell, chronic fatigue, vertigo, numbness, stroke, Parkinson's disease and nerve damage.

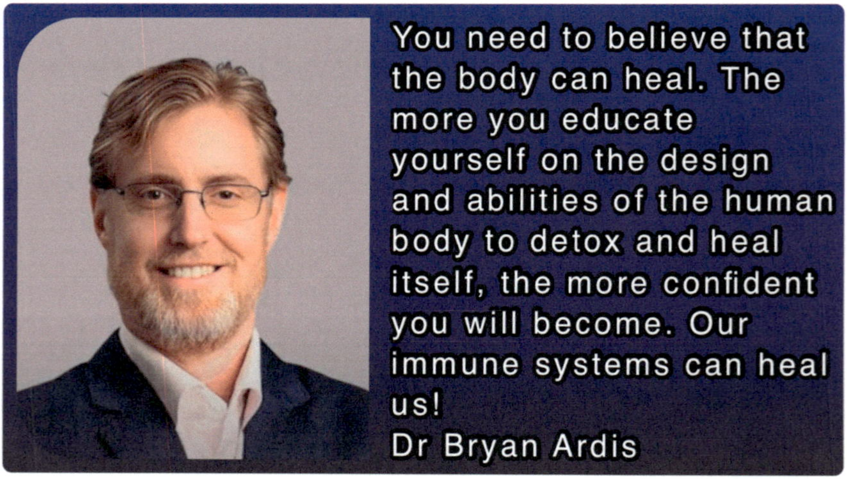

At the end of his book, Bryan outlines a wide range of suggestions to recover from long covid. These are often written from the perspective that this huge variety of symptoms might just be from snake toxins.

He lists five different tests you might ask for to check various covid long hauler health issues:

D-Dimer test for blood clots,

Troponin test for heart muscle inflammation,

Phospholipase A2, an enzyme linked to organ failure

Phosphodiesterase test, for a clotting enzyme

L-Amino Acid Assay Test which is recommended for couples suffering infertility and miscarriages. He matches these tests with specific suggestions about what might be used to remedy those issues. This appears to be a very concise, thorough and practical collection of suggested protocols. These are very valuable clues for sufferers and practitioners alike.

I would add these two tests to his list:

Live blood analysis for a direct view of the cells and any clumping or contamination

Full blood work from the pathology lab.

Essential oils:

Some dark field microscopists tell us that essential oils can help to clear nano-filaments. If anyone with a dark field microscope is keen to experiment with essential oils, Dr Ana Milhacea mentions 2 drops each of grapefruit, lemon, cinnamon, peppermint and oregano oil in veggie capsules, twice a day. This is not a recipe or a protocol, only an idea.

This is an adaptation of Dr Hildegarde Staninger's suggestion to clear unwanted tech from the blood: 2 drops each of grapefruit, lemon and cinnamon oils in an empty veggie capsule, twice a day.

Note that apparently grapefruit essential oils react badly with some medications.

If anyone with access to a dark field microscope to monitor their before and after results is keen to experiment with essential oils, they need a very high-quality oil. I have seen an extended list of oils appearing several times now in suggestions from various sources, which is encouraging: Grapefruit, lemon, lemon balm, cinnamon, peppermint, oregano, pine needle, rosemary and frankincense.

These would be a starter point for more research in this area It's interesting to note that natural oils like this can be very powerful, as seen in the fact that turpentine (made from the resin of certain pine trees) is the natural solvent for cleaning oil-based paint from brushes. In recent years many cleaning products have been based on orange and lemon oils. We know from our own kitchens that eucalyptus oil is great for removing those sticky labels from jars and appliances.

That's what we want: Something powerful enough to destroy strange new contamination and gentle enough not to damage our blood and organs.

Morgellons relief

An experienced microscopist spoke of a mixture of ingredients which may be useful to rub on Morgellons wounds to get relief:

Benzoin resinoid (this sounds a bit like an Asian

version of our own pine resin and is often used in natural perfumes.)

Lemon Oil

Grapefruit Oil

Neem Oil

Oregano Oil

Black Seed Oil

Mix equal parts of the oils and apply to the lesions.

Not Medical Advice

We have also had a report that an amateur microscopist looked at an itchy spot on his arm under the microscope and was horrified to see Morgellons fibres in there. He applied black salve, a powerful and controversial skin cancer remedy which I have used successfully several times. This drew the strange fibres out of the body into the thick black salve eschar.

Only people who can check the effects of what they are doing with live blood checks should experiment with completely unknown treatments without guidance. There is the chance that something they are doing makes the situation worse. This caution also applies to powered frequency devices like Rife and similar machines other than those mentioned here which have undergone more testing with nanotech contamination.

I am told by an experienced live blood microscopist that natural coherent frequencies like singing in harmony, tuning forks, singing bowls and gongs are beneficial to the blood. They don't remove the strange fairy light structures but they do help the red blood cells to separate from each other and flow better so blood function improves.

Ana Milhacea's suggestions for clearing out nano-filaments

Dr Ana Milhacea was almost a lone voice talking openly about this strange new contamination on many platforms from around 2022. She has written three books on the subject as a legacy to humanity which you can find in the links and references.

These are her main suggestions for the clearing of nano-micro technology from the blood from her book: Transhumanism – Overcoming the Global Depopulation Agenda.

'The work compiled in this book is my contribution for the survival of our species and the future of humanity'
Dr Ana Milhacea. 17 August 2024.

Looking at this huge line up, I believe this is a list that you and your naturopath might choose from, rather than a suggestion to use them all.

Calcium disodium EDTA microsomal from Global Healing - 2.5 droppers daily or as tolerated.

Stop taking EDTA if you get cramps.

Magnesium L-Threonate: 2 grams daily, if needed.

quality multi-mineral supplements each morning –

Dr. Tennant's® Restore: 1 scoop. If this is not available, substitute with a quality multi-mineral supplement each morning.

Chlorophyll: 1 tablespoon in filtered water.

(This detoxes and helps repair DNA.) Blue-green algae, spirulina, and coriander leaves (cilantro) are all helpful.

Neo 40 Professional: 1 daily. Helps the microbiome to dissolve graphene, helps circulation and heart function.

NAC: 1 gram daily - precursor to glutathione, detoxes metals and graphene.

Vitamin C: 8-10 grams daily or to gut tolerance. Used with EDTA this is an electron donor and chelates metals.

Humic and Fulvic Acid: 1.8 grams daily. This detoxes metals and graphene. It is shown to increase cellular electricity. (Ana suggests more, but I'm being cautious).

DMG (Dimethylglycine): 1 gram. This causes methyl groups to make more glutathione which detoxes graphene.

Nattokinase: 20.000 FU (fibrin units) daily.(1,000 milligams or l gram). This is several times more than the McCullough protocol. Ana tells us that this dissolves micro-clotting better than lower doses when viewed in live blood analysis. Use depending on patient need.

Methylene Blue: pharmaceutical grade - 50 mg daily. (According to Ana it dissolves rubbery clots.)

(I would tend to use BluZone 1% pharmaceutical grade, l drop per 4 kilos of body weight) or check the packaging.

Activated Charcoal: 500 mg daily. (.05 grams) Check the packaging for dosage.

Probiotics: daily. (take an hour after methylene-blue)

Malic Acid: 600 mg or 1 cap daily. (In the Moderna patent it is said to clear nanoparticles.)

Essential Oils: Grapefruit, lemon, cinnamon, peppermint and oregano: 2 drops each in (empty) veggie capsules daily.

Boron: 2 mg is in Restore already. If you do not take Dr. Tennant's® Restore, use boron.

Glutathione: The body's master antioxidant, detoxing and supporting immune function.

Dr Ana Milhacea's frontrunners for nanotechnology detox:

1 EDTA for eliminating metals used for biosensors and regenerating the red-blood-cell zeta-potential to prevent clotting.

2 High dose vitamin C for clot prevention and regeneration of electrical conductivity of the blood.

3 Methylene Blue as a clean-up for hydrogel and a powerful electron donor.

4 Essential oils, as mentioned to dissolve polymer plastics like polystyrene.

Again, she has a special mention for Plaquex to strengthen the cell membrane and Dr Tennant's

Restore because of his research on cellular health. It's available in Australia from desertcart.com.au

I believe we owe a huge debt of gratitude to Dr Ana Milhacea for sounding the alarm almost single handed, spear-heading this fledgeling movement, and formulating these ideas.

They give open minded practitioners starting points they can adapt depending on patient needs and results.

I would not want to embark on any program like this without naturopathic or other expert support and guidance.

A Simple Adaptation

I realised that in fact my own lovely naturopath Kirsty Bednar, Empower U Natural Health, had suggested a simplified version of this, which I did for a month, alongside other quality daily supplements. My live blood analysis following this in September 2025 was very promising, with free-flowing blood and very few nano-filaments.

This protocol is a perfect example of what we are trying to do with many of these treatments:

- Strengthen the organs of the body to work at an optimum level.
- Remove any nano structures and toxic metals from the blood and organs.
- Make sure they are gathered up by some sort of toxin binder, such as activated charcoal.
- Flush them harmlessly out of the body
- Replace beneficial minerals
- Oxygenate the body.

I started off with detoxing shakes each morning and afternoon using Metagenics Thermophase Detox for liver support, Metagenics G-Tox Express for kidneys, lymphatics and heavy metals. (They tasted pretty good whizzed up as a smoothie)

I did a second Global Healing liver cleanse, (I'm getting used to drinking strange concoctions) and then went on to:

1ml Global Healing microsomal Calcium Disodium EDTA
Take before sleep

(I take this in empty cellulose capsules which you can get from Miracle Products. Those of us with perfect teeth and zero metals in our mouths won't need this precaution. As EDTA pulls out metals, I wasn't taking any chances.)

1ml Global Healing Toxin Binder
Take the following day, 20 minutes before breakfast

This formula includes activated charcoal which makes sure that what you have pulled out of the tissues is picked up and actually leaves the body. It looks weird but tastes fine.

1-2 teaspoons Vitamin C powder, in water, to bowel tolerance.
Daily.

I used Eden Health Foods Wild C and blended it in the Nutri-Bullet type blender with water and an orange. It tasted great.

Bowel tolerance means that you flush out the system so well you might have to rush to the bathroom. Be prepared.

HOCATT

This is Hyperbaric Ozone Carbonic Acid Transdermal Technology. I'm sure the units vary but if you can find a clinic with one of these pod-like units, this has been recommended as a therapeutic to clear and sweat out toxins and heavy metals. It offers ozone, steam, light therapy, frequency specific microcurrents that can be tuned to 100 ailments and far infra-red to heat the body and stimulate blood flow. It sounds amazing.

It may be helpful in the clearing of nanoparticles, but again I would use caution with the frequencies, making sure that the clinic you use is aware of the new contamination in our blood and its interactions with the body.

Hyperbaric Oxygen Therapy (HBOT)

According to Dr Eric Berg, when we breathe normally, we only take in 21% oxygen. With the pressurised hyperbaric oxygen chamber that percentage of oxygen goes up to nearly 100% and it is taken up by tissues and blood. It drives a high amount of concentrated oxygen into injured and oxygen starved tissues and stimulates your own healing stem cells by 800%.

This is beneficial for a huge array of ailments, including helping to clear nano-micro-filaments and nano-tech from the blood. We have an anecdotal story of a woman who had live blood analysis and a disappointing amount of nanotech in her blood before visiting a retreat overseas. She received hyperbaric oxygen therapy on most days during the retreat and her blood was seen to be very much improved on her return, even after many hours in the air.

Ultimate Parasite Cleanse

After you've done a colon cleanse and three liver cleanses, you're ready for the Ultimate Parasite Cleanse metal and chemical detox and a final Liver Cleanse to clear the last of the toxins.

These protocols are designed by Maria Crisler and include beginner, intermediate and advanced cleanses. Dr Ria and Dr Ed Group are a part of this important collaboration.

The Ultimate parasite cleanse was released in April 2025.

It was formulated to help clear the body of natural and synthetic parasites and contamination of all sorts.

We live in extremely polluted and unprecedented times and I believe that investing money and focus on these cleanses are a better option than the possible effects of having increasingly polluted blood and toxicity in our bodies. I do recommend that you find an open-minded naturopath or health professional to support you through the process if you can.

Find the PDF at Buymeacoffee Longhaulers Evolving Solutions behind a very modest paywall. With thanks to Dr Ria Hayes.

Most of the products are from Dr Ed Group's company, Global Healing which are of an extremely high quality, but I will list them here:

Cellcore:	Para 1
Global Healing:	Microsomal EDTA
Global Healing:	InsuLess
Global Healing:	Paratrex 2
Global Healing:	Toxin Binder
Global Healing	Oxy Powder
Global Healing:	Supercharged C60
Global Healing:	Ozonated Activated charcoal
Covilife 12	Ivermectin
Global Healing	Fermented digestive enzymes
Global Healing	Latero Flora

Not all supplements are equal.

I am being very specific with recommendations so you have the best chance of healing quickly and effectively. I would be confident buying Ivermectin from this brand after a recommendation from these professionals. Great news for Australians, there is a new Australian Stockist for Global Healing. Many of their products are now available from Sage Wellbeing, *sagewellbeing.com.au*

Other supplements may be good but may not be tested for this new purpose.

The ULTIMATE PARASITE CLEANSE BEGINNER PROTOCOL

Ensure you fast for 18-24 hours once weekly

AT LEAST 3 GLOBAL HEALING LIVER CLEANSES (one 6 day and 2x Two Day)
NEED TO BE COMPLETED PRIOR TO ANY PARASITE DETOX
TO OPEN UP ELIMINATION PATHWAYS.

2 Weeks on 2 Weeks off; taper back as needed to manage any Detox Symptoms

Wake Up and take on an Empty Stomach:
2 Capsules Cellcore Para 1
(**OPTIONA**L 1ml Global Healing Microsomal EDTA Morning or Evening **EVERY OTHER DAY**)

Morning 10-30 mins **BEFORE MEAL**: 5 drops InsuLess
2ml Global Healing Paratrex 2 Microsomal

1 Hour Post Meal 1ml Global Healing Toxin Binder

Lunch 10-30 mins **BEFORE MEAL**: 2-5 drops InsuLess
2 Capsules Fermented Digestive Enzymes with food

Late Afternoon 2 Capsules Latero Flora

Dinner 10-30 mins **BEFORE MEAL:** 5 drops InsuLess
2ml Global Healing Paratrex 2 Microsomal

1 Hour Post Meal 1ml Global Healing Toxin Binder

Evening Bedtime on an Empty Stomach:
3-5 Capsules Oxy Powder

For additional binding to manage Herxheimer symptoms you can add Supercharged C60 or Ozonated Activated Charcoal **2 hours away from meds/supplements** taken the same time as Toxin Binder

Ivermectin 12mg Covilife12 from our trusted supplier for 5 years delivered to 1000's patients worldwide can be added during your 2 weeks on protocol. Take with fat for better absorption.

Use Code RIA15 for 15% DISCOUNT For All Global Healing Products

These protocols are suggestions. Always check with your practitioner before taking any supplements. We do not intend to treat, diagnose, or cure; but we have developed these protocols to assist you with your detoxification journey and to educate on product usage. Please discontinue use of supplementation or protocol should you experience aggressive detoxification symptoms. Please adjust where needed according to your detoxification reaction journey.

I do not take any commission from any treatment recommended)

We are in a new situation here and owe it to ourselves to use the best tools we can find.

Global Healing Complete Body Cleanse program

This appears to be the best all-in-one, state-of-the-art cleansing program to restore optimal organ function. The company makes no promises about nano tech removal, but the all-important oral EDTA and Toxin Binder products which work on this are included in the line-up.

This whole process starts at the very beginning with a colon cleanse and steps you right through the complete protocol. It's likely to take 4 months, depending on how much break you take between detoxes. You may have a detoxing headache or feel tired but it will help if you drink plenty of filtered water and exercise through the process. You should eat fresh, healthy organic foods and it's likely that you'll have more energy, enhanced immunity, mental clarity and general wellbeing when you've completed it.

This is not a cheap process by any means, but it appears to be the most comprehensive, high quality supplement-based healing package that you can undertake with minimal supervision if you have to. I discovered when doing their liver cleanses that the instructions are wonderfully simple and straightforward. You also have access to support by email and phone support if you have to undertake this journey alone.

Tony Pantalleresco and the Anti Nano bucket

I thought I had collected all the solutions I could when I chanced upon Tony Pantalleresco. Watching him talking while he made the bucket reminded me of Doc Brown, the eccentric scientist from the film, 'Back to the Future'. Most of us remember that Doc Brown actually achieved amazing things in the film.

Tony's rudimentary website includes lots of research of various kinds and the aim of the bucket and various other devices is to create a magnetic field that will disrupt this self-assembling nanotech so it turns off and the body can finally get rid of it.

This principle makes sense to me. Tony also repeats my own concern that other frequency devices, The 'Rife' machine, or Hulda Clark's parasite zapper, which seem to be otherwise useful and safe when used carefully, may make this nano-technology contamination worse. Elana Freeland, a highly respected author in this field, also mentions Tony Pantalleresco's work in her book 'The Geoengineered Transhuman'.

It seems that within a few minutes of turning on the anti-nano device and immersing the feet, the nano tech is pulled out of the skin and begins to collect in a sparkly scum on top of the solution.

I am tempted to say, 'Don't try this at home' … certainly not unless you feel confident. And always remember that electricity and water don't mix.

I have included as many videos of him and the bucket in the links as I can in the possibility of inspiring further research in this area.

E:OO

EBOO (Extra-Corporeal Blood Oxygenation, Ozonation and Filtration Blood-Cleansing).

As at July 2026, qualified EBOO practitioners are still a very rare commodity. Evolve Clinics are based in England, Palma and Cyprus and a beautiful new EBOO clinic, Helix Institute has opened in Auckland, New Zealand and I am hopeful that more specialist clinics may open up soon.

I believe we need them. Clotting has become such an issue since 2022 that rubbery clots of up to half a metre long sometimes block the lines and have to be pulled out by hand before they can continue the process. Smaller clots can also be seen as even previously healthy bodies of people in their prime have become overwhelmed with sludgy toxins. These are directly related to the nano-filaments, hydrogel and other impurities in our blood.

The sad fact is that unless we can check and monitor our blood on a regular basis, we don't know if these nano-filaments are multiplying, clotting our blood, especially when we can see chemtrails and other potential contamination in the sky.

The EBOO treatment uses a patented blood-filtration process to physically remove moulds, pesticides, dead and diseased cells, cholesterol, spike-proteins,clots and heavy metals.

It takes 60 minutes during which time your blood will receive 60 litres of pure oxygen and ozone as needed, along with filtration. You sit back in a comfortable chair and have two cannulas and lines attached. One is a draw line taking blood *out* of the body and the other one is putting it back *in*. Impurities, inflammation and debris in the blood is left in a waste jar along the way. The drug Heperin is used carefully in the process to keep the blood flowing freely without clotting and clogging up the lines.

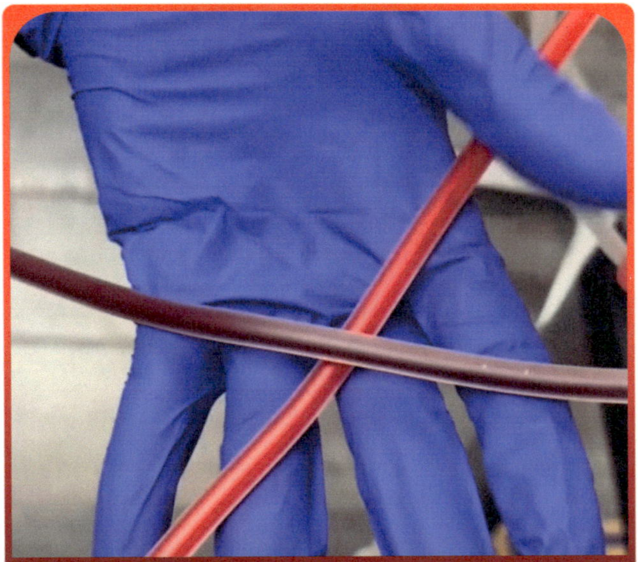

EBOO (extra corporeal blood oxygenation and ozonation therapy). The dark line is the blood leaving the body, the bright red line is the filtered and oxygenated blood ready to be returned into the body.

The 'old' blood straight from the body is often dark red and lumpy while the 'filtered and oxygenated blood' is bright red, clear and healthy. This is an amazing treatment, but even this is not a once-and-for-all answer. Other cleansing options should be used on a regular basis.

Clinical Chelation Therapy

EDTA (ethylene-diamene-tetra-acetic-acid) acts very quickly, is much more specialised and involves injecting a chelator into the bloodstream. There are a variety of chelators you might need. The main ones attach to heavy metals in the blood. Once attached, they escort the unwanted metals through the kidneys and they're flushed out of the body in the urine.

This is one of Dr Ana Milhacea's procedures in her US clinic, and she describes the blood being clear, healthy and flowing freely in a few sessions. This is monitored carefully with live blood analysis before and after treatments.

These clinical treatments are more drastic measures than the other protocols but if you are suffering badly after the covid shots without other medical diagnosis or explanation, this might be a worth-while option for you. Clinics are very few and far between so, you may need to factor travel and accommodation into your costs.

Green Laser Therapies

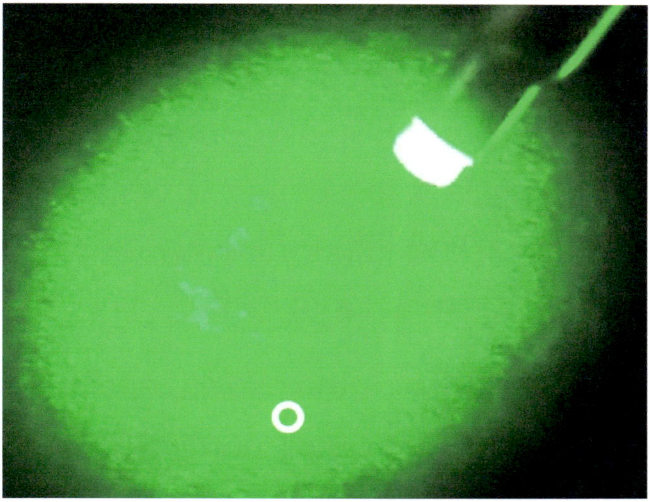

A Trip to Auckland

Towards what I thought was the end of my journey, still metaphorically feeling my way through thick bushland, researching and putting clues together, the Great Spirit suddenly seemed to take a real interest and orchestrated an amazing experience.

I had been on David Nixon's international microscopy chat group and Zoom meetings for months. It's very interesting and I learned many things, but my own focus was always not so much 'What are these things?' 'Where do they come from?' or 'What are they doing?' All of which are important, but, 'How do we get rid of them?'

Then one day a voice spoke up and talked about an Auckland clinic with queues of people lining up outside the door and I heard the words 'green laser therapy. I had to see it for myself.

I live in country New South Wales, and a few days and two plane rides later, half wondering if I was on a wild goose chase, I arrived at the small Auckland lab of an experienced microscopist and avid researcher I'll call Mark. We talked briefly about the array of fascinating microscopes, bright violet and green lights and the urgency of this work, before heading off across town to another clinic: The Helix Institute, 56 Barry's Point Road, Takapuna.

This beautiful clinic, is probably New Zealand's only clinic offering EBOO, Weber green laser and other new high-tech modalities. Mark took a finger-prick sample of my blood which had looked so good a few weeks before. It seemed to have suffered from something since then and didn't look good at all. This was a bit of a shock.

The lovely nurse took me into a gorgeous room with brand new white suede-leather lounge chairs. She put a cannula (an entry point into the vein) into my arm and took a test tube of before blood before inserting a fluorescent green laser optical fibre so

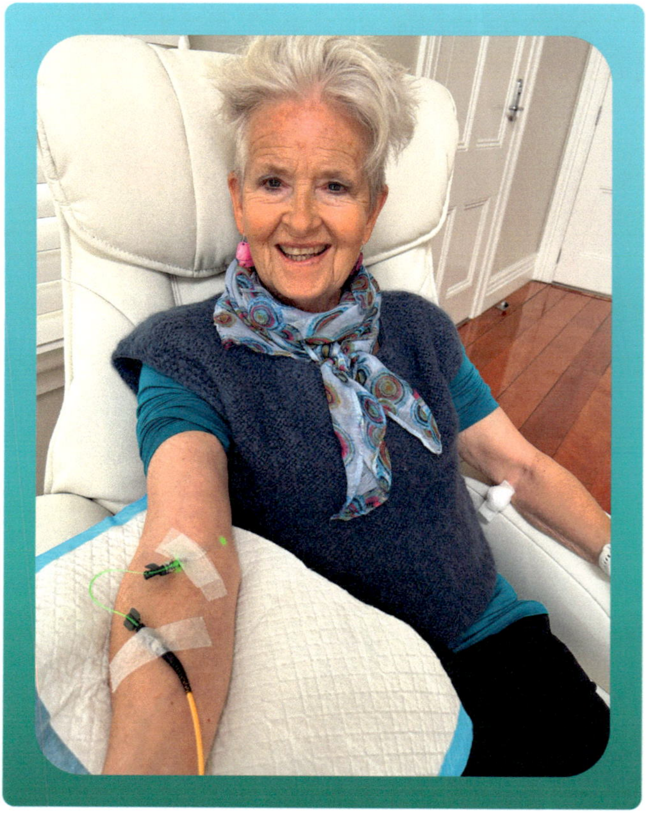

bright you could see it shining from inside my arm. It didn't hurt at all. I relaxed with peaceful music for 25 minutes before she came back to remove the green laser and take another test tube of blood for the after sample.

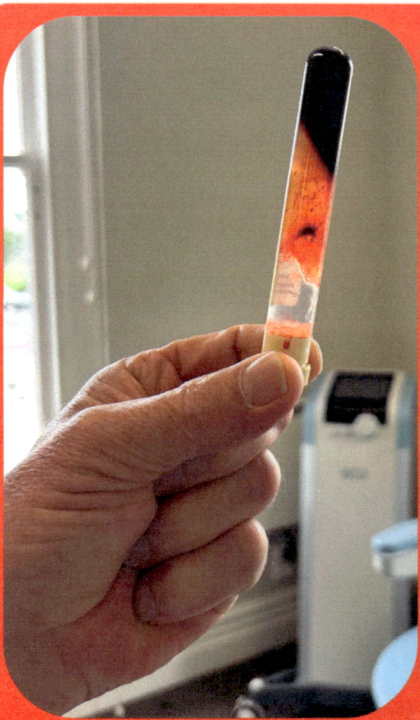

Top left:
Clotted blood
before the
intravenous
green laser
treatment:

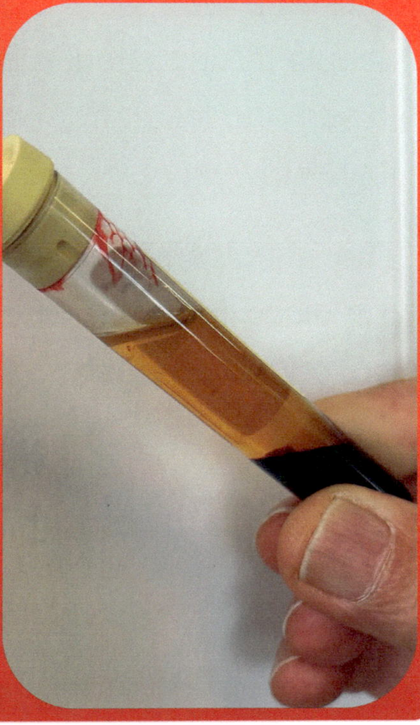

Lower right:
After the
treatment
Blood
clear and
flowing.

These blood samples were left to stand for 30 minutes. This is the blood's normal coagulation and healing process and is no longer active after half an hour. They were both put in the centrifuge (like a tiny spin dryer) to separate the plasma from the red blood cells.

As you can see, the before sample was so thick the plasma made a white rubbery plug in the test tube. This was another shock. It's one thing to listen to people talking about rubbery clots but quite another to see one taken from a small vial of my own blood. It was my very own rubbery clot.

The after sample was clear and free flowing and the blood from the 'after' finger-prick blood sample looked much better.

My very own rubbery clot
Wendy Danel
https://youtube.com/shorts/BevsRWLZJ3w?si=cgpGQRIDH61X6YIT

It was quietly mind blowing.

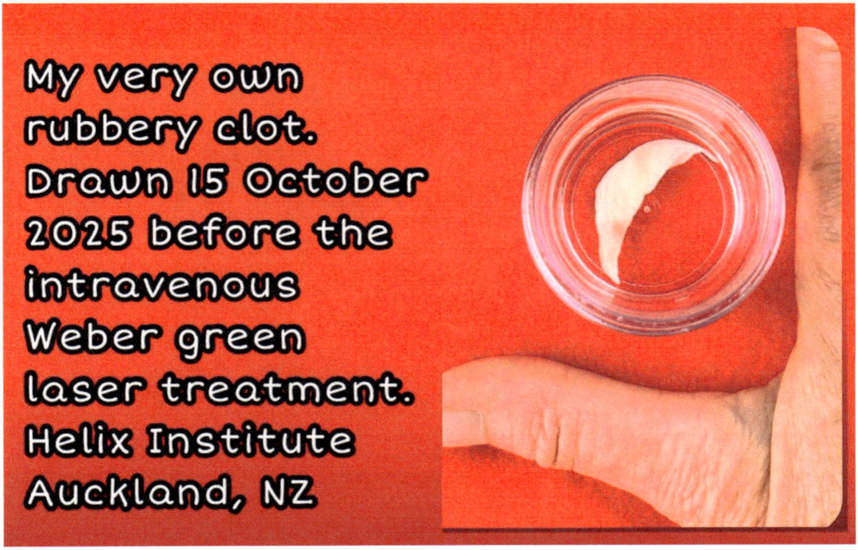

Mark drove us back to his own lab and I began to understand the significance of the green lights I had seen before. I am told that these are three times as strong as the intravenous low level light therapy and about 80% as effective. The big advantage is that they can be shined on the delicate skin on the inside of the wrist or the back of the hand. They are even portable.

Some people may feel nothing from this treatment, some may feel a tingling, warmth, or even euphoria due to increased oxygen coming to the brain. If people start to feel uncomfortable, the light is moved further away to lessen the effect. During a half-hour treatment the blood circulates the body around thirty times and, according to Mark, the Weber green laser is also helpful for varicose veins and Morgellons lesions.

Low level laser light therapy

So how do these colourful lasers work their magic?

Most of us are familiar with the effects of normal lasers. We've seen how they can cut intricate shapes into wood and steel, zap an unwanted blemish off the skin or perform precision eye surgery in a way that's impossible with physical tools.

Low level or Weber laser therapy is used to promote healing and restoration of the tissues. Finely tuned light energy and frequency is transformed into energy that stimulates the body for various functions.

Red, blue, and yellow low level laser therapies can be used to improve a very wide variety of debilitating chronic issues but for this strange, new and elusive blood issue, it seems that green light penetrates deeper into the tissues and takes the prize.

The Auckland team worked for months using themselves as guinea pigs, to find the right combination of light wave and frequency. It's not a simple matter. Many other variations may make the condition worse and the green lasers must remain tuned and fixed at exactly the same frequency to give benefit.

Mark uses the non-invasive laser on himself every day, five minutes in the morning and ten minutes in the afternoon, along with a whole lemon and ginger drink, grounding, a few drops of hydrogen peroxide in water and iodine to maintain health in these strange contaminated times.

ELFET/Tri-Vortex Green Laser Therapy

Back in Australia, keen to learn a little more about the Weber green laser I had experienced, I learned that an Australian practitioner was using a green laser therapy and getting great results.

A brief conversation made it clear that, while this therapist also used a green laser, and was getting repeatable success, this was a completely different technology:

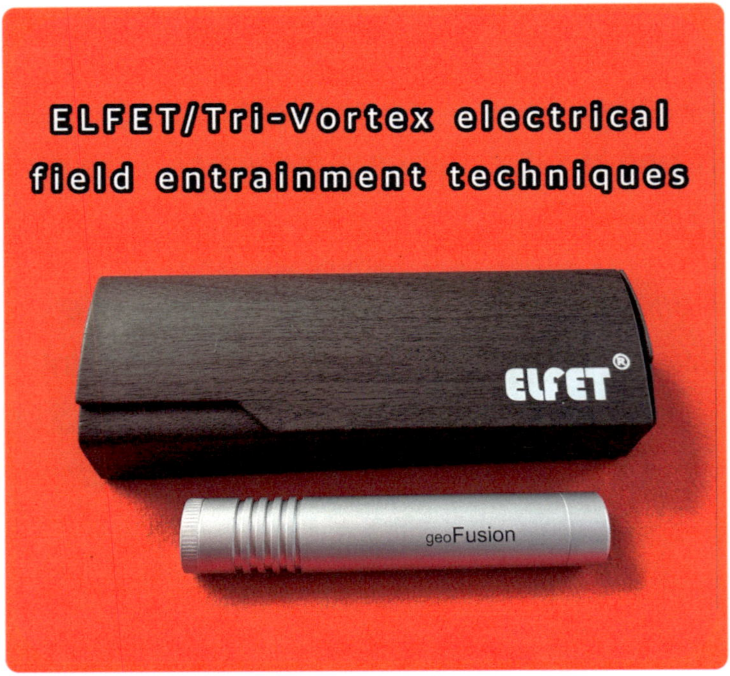

ELFET/Tri-Vortex is a chemical-free, bio-mimicry-based process that imparts naturally optimized geometric resonances into materials. It uses proprietary frequency techniques of converting geometries into sound equivalents and incorporates bespoke software developed over decades, to create subtle energy products.

This unique system offers a huge variety of practical, visionary results in many fields, notably water structuring, pain relief, agriculture, bee-keeping and animal husbandry.

These are geometries that you will find in the creation processes throughout the biological world. The main focus for us at this time is that this technology serves as a reminder to the body of how nature creates optimally.

It seems to me that many therapies work on 'nudging' the body in some way to do what it needs to do. In their different ways this might be said of homeopathy, acupuncture, Bowen therapy, and even black salve. I believe this therapy could be thought of in the same way as it reminds the body of its strongest optimum self so it can rid itself of this new contamination.

A few days and a couple of conversations later a small, slim torch-like ELFET/Tri-Vortex green laser and some water structuring discs arrived in the mail. This laser treatment works on a longer timeline than the other laser, but has the big advantage of being battery powered and portable enough to fit in your pocket. The main precaution is not to shine it into your eyes.

My plan was to do live blood analysis with my normal practitioner *before* and then *after* several days. I started on 27th November 2025. As suggested, I held the laser directly onto the pulse point of my inner right wrist and muscle tested that this was the optimum spot for me to place the laser. I personally started off needing 23 minutes in that position morning and afternoon. (This is quite a lot. Some people are much more sensitive and need less time.) My muscle testing (and a consultation with my psychic reader) shows me that two weeks later my blood was over 70% improved and the laser treatment time I needed was down to 11 minutes, morning and evening. I muscle tested these treatment times and improvements in my blood every day and found that the times I needed the Tri-Vortex laser became shorter, and shorter, while my blood muscle tested better and better over the weeks.

By early January 2026, Just six weeks after I had started the treatment, I muscle tested that my blood was clear. I don't think this is a permanent result as we are still being re-contaminated in various ways.

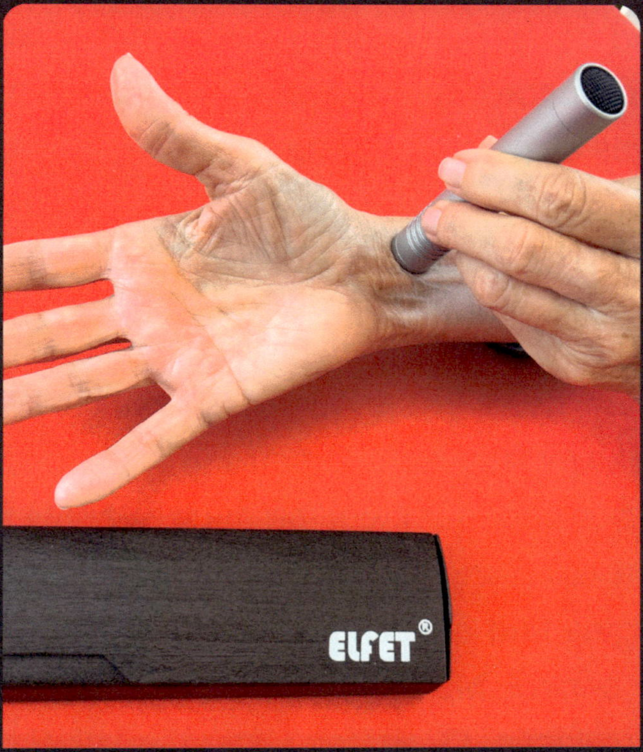

Using the ELFET Tri-Vortex laser

We have to think in terms of ongoing precautions, but it was very exciting all the same.

It was time for another trip to Newcastle to check the blood.

My blood at this test was as good as it had ever been. I would have liked it to be perfect but only a couple of filaments could be seen and the blood was flowing freely. Considering our recontamination and the fact I hadn't used the laser for a couple of weeks, this was an outstanding result.

Keeping Score

I had personally used four different strategies one after the other in the 18 months since I first saw these shiny fairy light filaments in my blood. I visited my psychic reader friend on my way home from the 'final' reading and she was able to tell me that all four strategies had actually worked well to keep things under control. Methylene Blue, and the EDTA/ toxin binder/vitamin C strategy were relatively cheap, simple and effective. Both of these were thought to be best cycled to allow the body a break for a couple of days.

The Weber green laser in Auckland was a spectacular success, and of great benefit, especially if you happen to live in New Zealand. The Elfet Tri-Vortex laser is my treatment of choice. My psychic friend reported that, used properly, it was 100% beneficial. (I checked this bold statement with her very carefully). It's also safe for use on children, with the reminder that it is not a toy and should not be left with them to use on their own.

After the first clearing, I believe that for me about 6 minutes, morning and evening, would be enough to keep the contamination at bay and the blood circulating happily. Although more expensive than the first options I particularly like the fact that this treatment doesn't require us to take extra substances, other than basic vitamins, on an ongoing basis. Other treatments could be used occasionally, if wished and I do believe that regular liver cleansing is much more important than most of us realised.

Treatment of dental anaesthetics

One of the consistent sources of nanotech contamination we have found in these strange times are dental anaesthetics. Many medical preparations are also suspect but unless we have perfect teeth, dental anaesthetics are hard to avoid.

Another extraordinary feature of the ELFET/Tri-Vortex technology is their custom chamber, which can be used to remove nanotechnology from things like vials of dental anaesthetic and other medications.

Vials of dental anaesthetic were put into the ELFET/Tri-Vortex chamber for 24 hours, then sent to four independent kinesiologists along with untreated vials, for blind testing. All four kinesiologists found the Tri-Vortex treated vials to be safe to use, and the untreated vials to be unsafe.

As at 2026, most dentists are unaware of this.

Cancer

Cancer rates have risen alarmingly in the post covid era. It's unsure whether this is a direct reaction to the covid shots weakening our immune systems, shedding, parasites, the lack of oxygen in the blood leading cells to clump together or a combination of all of them. There may be many things that are directly contributing to what are accurately being described as turbo-cancers.

In the world of conventional cancer treatments there are recognised patterns, predictable ages of diagnosis and estimated life expectancy. Whatever we think of these predictions, in the years since 2022 a range of bigger, faster and more aggressive cancers has changed the landscape. Types of cancer that had been growing slowly in people in their seventies were suddenly seen growing fast in previously healthy people in their twenties and thirties. 'Conventional' treatments like chemotherapy and radiation were failing.

I have posted a collection of natural cancer treatments on Facebook for many years, updating them over trime. I included them in 'Detox after Covid and Thrive.' and make no apology for including them, updated yet again, here. These insights and leads may be life-saving for some readers or their friends and family, especially as it's even more important to act fast in the post-covid era. It's important for us all to realise how censored and demonised simple cancer cures have been for nearly 100 years.

Dr Max Gerson's therapy has been curing people of cancer (and other diseases) consistently since the thirties. The treatment is mostly veggie juices and coffee enemas to alkalize and cleanse the system.

In 1952 Dr Raymond Kaiser, Head of the National Cancer Institute, on seeing Gerson's meticulous records of many cures of advanced cancer cases, said, 'Sometimes these European Refugees come over to America and want to make a splash so they go ahead and cure cancer.'

The Gerson Institute in San Diego is still a thriving hub of knowledge and healing world-wide.

In 1934, after many years of work, gifted scientist Royal Raymond Rife conducted an experiment at the University of Southern California using targeted electromagnetic frequencies to kill cancer. 16 terminally ill cancer patients were cured painlessly within 4 months. A grand dinner was held in his honour.

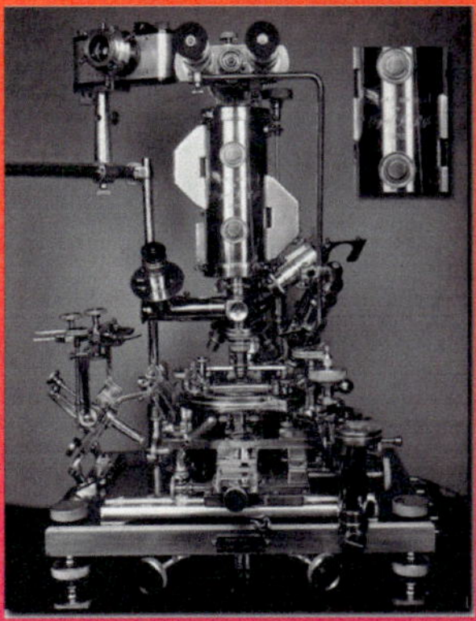

'Due to the unique properties of the Rife Universal Microscope, the researchers noted various colors associated with different microbes. Rife and his researchers discovered that these microbes could be destroyed by shattering them with the exact frequency that resonated with each type. Rife called the lethal frequency that shattered a microbe, bacteria or virus, its Mortal Oscillatory Rate (MOR).'
Dr Steven Ross PhD

The medical industry then began the systematic destruction of Rife's groundbreaking technology, his labs, his records, the equipment he had made and Rife himself. He died a broken man.

Check out Black Salve on YouTube which is very effective for skin cancers. I have used this myself several times and it worked exactly as shown. I suggest you try it first on an area of skin that isn't so prominent, like your arm, while you check how it works. (Link at the back of the book)

Harry Hoxey was curing cancer for decades with recipes derived from Native American recipes and the work continues under the name of the Hoxey Bio Medical Centre.

Laetrile or amygdalin for B17 (from apricot kernels and other bitter stone-fruit seeds) was proved in tests by highly regarded Dr Kanematsu Sugiura at the Sloane-Kettering institute to be one of the most effective anti-cancer treatments ever tested on mice. Then it was systematically discredited by that same organisation and later outlawed in the US.

One of the longest-lived communities in the world, the Hunza, has loads of apricots in their diet and prizes the kernels highly. A man's wealth is counted in apricot trees. Cancer is virtually unknown. In 1974, Dr John Richardson wrote 'A World without Cancer, the story of B17' with his good friend, G. Edward Griffin who is the official author. Global Healing has a quality B17 which is good for prevention as well as treatment.

Dr Eric Berg has many great YouTube clips on cancer and has an excellent PDF on suitable diets.

Dr Berg's Five diet strategies for cancer care: https://drbrg.co/4om43oQ

Check out 'Chris beat Cancer' for the story of a young man who, cured his colon cancer naturally and has taught others how to do the same for many years. His latest 'Square One' program is a wonderful guide that anyone can make their own.

In the post-covid era I would 100% add Ivermectin and Fenbendazole or natural parasite remedies to this protocol. Dr William Makis has described hundreds of successful case studies using these anti-parasitics on his Substack.

Dr Stanislaw Burzynski discovered that people with cancer lack certain peptides and pioneered what he called anti-neoplaston cancer treatment in the 80s.

The Burzynski clinic in Texas specialises in treating children's brain cancers with no toxic side effects and a significant percentage of complete recoveries. He was harassed by the Texas Medical Board for three decades for continuing this life saving work.

Check the documentary of the same name: Burzynski

Cancer is a disease of toxicity coupled with vitamin and mineral deficiencies, oxygen deficiency, (singlet oxygen is especially important) and dehydration so the body can't throw it off any longer.

'Cancer cells and many other imbalances cannot survive in a hydrated, oxygenated, alkaline environment. It's that simple.' Ed McCabe: Flood Your Body with Oxygen. 'No disease, including cancer, can exist in an alkaline environment.' Otto Warburg, 1931 Nobel Prize Winner for cancer discovery.

Andreas Moritz explains what cancer is doing in the body. It gives clarity on why these changes are needed

Cancer is Not Trying to Kill You. It is Trying to Save You
https://youtu.be/r18OHoT5Q7o?si=3kO-63M4xlqRuwKp

Check out 'The Truth about Cancer' by Ty and Charlene Bollinger. On YouTube, Rumble and the website. Steep yourself in this information to really GET that it's real and possible.

'Cancer Decoded' is another wonderful resource by Jonathon Otto and dozens of knowledgeable guest speakers.

Find it on the Brighteon website.
www.brighteon.com/

How to stay healthy? Do some exercise you enjoy every day. Stay off the sugar, processed foods, fried stuff, seed oils, grains, dairy and alcohol. Eat raw organic whenever possible.

Enjoy lots of deep breathing, good air, raw salads, wheatgrass and organic veggie juices with the live plant nutrients still in them.

Drink filtered water, often with lemon juice and celtic salt to alkalize the system. Take an oxygen/mineral supplement, Vitamin D, C, CoQ10, magnesium, omega 3, iodine and B vitamins … And throw in a few of those apricot kernels for good measure …

If you are already there and have had a diagnosis:

- Stay calm. Make sure you are exercising every day. Go raw vegan organic with loads of juicing, little fruit, mostly veggies, and clear your environment of as many toxins as possible while you decide what to do.
- Colonic hydrotherapy sessions to clean out the large intestine would be of great benefit now.
- Meditate.
- DON'T let them rush you into chemo treatments and surgery.
- DON'T let them frighten you.
- Stay calm.
- Do your research carefully. You have many options.
- Choose the path that's right for you.
- Consider a naturopath or holistic practitioner

who has seen people in your position recover and believes you can too.

- Make a diary of every bit of progress and healing and be grateful and appreciative of every step in the right direction.

Your faith in your own recovery is paramount and you need to find a practitioner who believes in you.

One of the most consistently outspoken and dedicated Doctors of the post covid era is Czech-born Canadian Dr William Makis. He is a cancer doctor with an impressive number of degrees and a broad range of experience. He developed a highly targeted form of cutting-edge cancer treatment using tiny amounts of radiation with pin point precision.

The success of his treatment led to his clinic being sabotaged by the Canadian government and he found himself free enough from the system to speak out.

He has been treating people with repurposed drugs for two years and has had amazing and repeated success with previously hopeless cases either when the drugs are used alone or with targeted conventional treatments. Dr Makis posts details of successful treatments using these protocols on his Substack on most days.

They are clear, specific, and detailed enough that it seems sufferers have nothing to lose by trying these remedies. Many of the protocols include Ivermectin. An anti-parasitic drug, Ivermectin has been used millions of times in humans and animals over many years and has been found to be very successful against turbo cancers.

As at the second half of 2025, we believe this successful and virtually harmless anti-parasitic may have been tampered with to make it less effective. We have to be very careful of the brand and quality we choose.

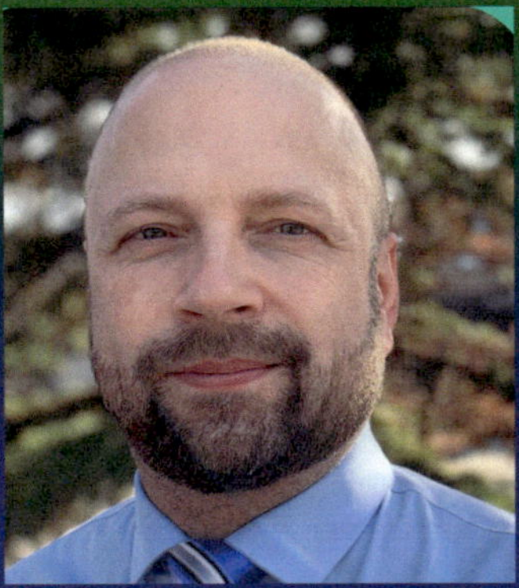

> 'There may be a parasitic component to cancer. A lot of anti-parasitics are actually effective against cancer. It isn't just Ivermectin. For example, Fenbendazol, artemisia (sweet wormwood), black walnut, and Praziquantel are also having success.
> Why is that?'
> Dr William Makis MD

There is a Telegram group called Fenbendazole and Ivermectin which has a vast wealth of information, hands on knowledge and feedback on these products.

A suitable dose for a major cancer might be

Ivermectin: 1 milligram per kilo of bodyweight per day. 7 days a week, for three months.

Half a milligram per kilo of bodyweight might be enough for a smaller cancer.

These doses work well for those on conventional treatments and even reduce the unpleasant side effects of chemotherapy.

Arthritis, fibromyalgia and rheumatoid arthritis can be treated with even smaller doses.

It is usually combined with Fenbendazol, the vetinerary anti-parasitic and the almost identical Mebendazol which is FDA (Food and Drug Administration, U.S.) approved for humans and has an excellent safety profile.

Mebendazole: A suitable starting dose for a major cancer might be 1,000 miligrams (1 gram) per day, 6 days on, one day off.

Half a gram per day would be a good starting dose for a smaller cancer.

A contact gave me a small bottle of pure Ivermectin. In early 2026 a friend told me that his mother had cancer. I shared all the information I had and gave him the bottle. In May 2026 he called me to say she was completely clear. She had started to feel better the moment she took the Ivermectin. Wendy Daniel

Dr William Makis MD
Protocol for Cancer

PHARMACYIN USA

IVERMECTIN DOSAGE

LOW DOSE	MEDIUM DOSE	HIGH DOSE	VERY HIGH DOSE
≤ 0.5mg/kg	1.0mg/kg	2.0mg/kg	≥ 2.5mg/kg
Cancers in remission Strong family history Genetic predisposition Prophylaxis	Starting dose for most cancers	Dose for very aggressive cancers (leukemia, pancreas, brain cancers)	Extensive metastatic disease Extremely poor prognosis Brain cancers?
No long term side effects	No long term side effects	No long term side effects	Possible short term & transient visual effects
Dr.Tess Lawrie reported a case of Stage 3 Ovarian Cancer, treated with chemo and 12mg of IVM per day, Ca125 dropped 288 to 22 after 2 months. Tumor vanished.	Dr. Shankara Chetty reported a 70 yo prostate ca patient with PSA 89, placed on 45mg IVM per day, after two months, PSA dropped from 89.1 to 10.9. IVM given in combination with Lactoferrin.	Dr. Allan Landrito had a Stage 4 gallbladder patient who took 2mg/kg/day for 14 months (cancer disappeared)	Dr.Shankara Chetty had a patient on 2.5mg/kg/day with no side effects

FENBENDZOLE DOSAGE

LOW DOSE	MEDIUM DOSE	HIGH DOSE	VERY HIGH DOSE
222mg 3x per week	222mg/day (6 days a week)	444mg/day (6 days a week)	888mg or 1000mg/day (6 days a week)
Cancers in remission Strong family history Genetic predisposition Prophylaxis	Starting dose for most cancers Weight < 200lb	mRNA Turbo Cancer Aggressive Cancers Stage 4 Weight 200+ lb	Extensive metastatic disease Extremely poor prognosis
Check liver function & kidney function	Check liver function & kidney function	Check liver function & kidney function	Check liver function & kidney function
222mg Fenbendazole 3 days on, 4 days off(panacur C) Vitamin E 800 IU/ day Curcumin 600mg/day CBD oil 25mg/day	Taken with/after meal Milk Thistle 250mg twice a day with food (liver support)	Taken with/after meal Milk Thistle 250mg twice a day with food (liver support)	Max 30-50mg/kg/day for 5 days (very rarely used in this dose range)

One of hundreds of 2025 testimonies was from a 47-year-old Australian woman with stage 4 advanced gastric cancer and metastases in the liver showing that the cancer had spread. In other words, she was in dire straits.

He started her on

Ivermectin, 1.5 milligrams per kilo per day
Fenbendazole 1.5 gams per day
CBD oil 100 milligrams per day
Melatonin 300 milligrams per day.

After 2 months, the metastases were gone. This is not medical advice but for entertainment purposes only.
There are thousands of testimonials like this on these two sites alone over two years. It is ironic that Dr Makis fled communist Czechoslovakia and came to Canada with his parents in the belief that it was a free country, yet in recent years he has has to defend his medical licence against an authority with an agenda.

This is a very familiar and heartbreaking story for doctors and scientists making real headway for the good of humanity.

The fact that these turbo cancers seem to be reduced so easily and quickly with these anti parasitic medicines is a real bonus in these challenging times.

Chris Beat Cancer. The Square One Program

As a backdrop for the new and aggressive cancers, we have Chris Wark's Square One program, which offers a wealth of knowledge about the best diet and lifestyle options for cancers generally. Having cured himself from colon cancer after an initial surgery in his twenties, Chris has guided many thousands of people to achieve the same results for themselves. In the process he has gained a detailed perspective of the challenges and strategies that have worked for people. His Square One Program puts it all together in a relatable package that helps people make the beneficial diet plans work with their lifestyle.
This protocol can be used as a foundation to the Makis recommendations for maximum effect.

This is not medical advice.
Turbo cancers and repurposed drugs

Dr John Campbell talks to Dr William Makis
https://youtu.be/0gIYQCjB_NU?si=dN-wMR4Na7GAx7nb

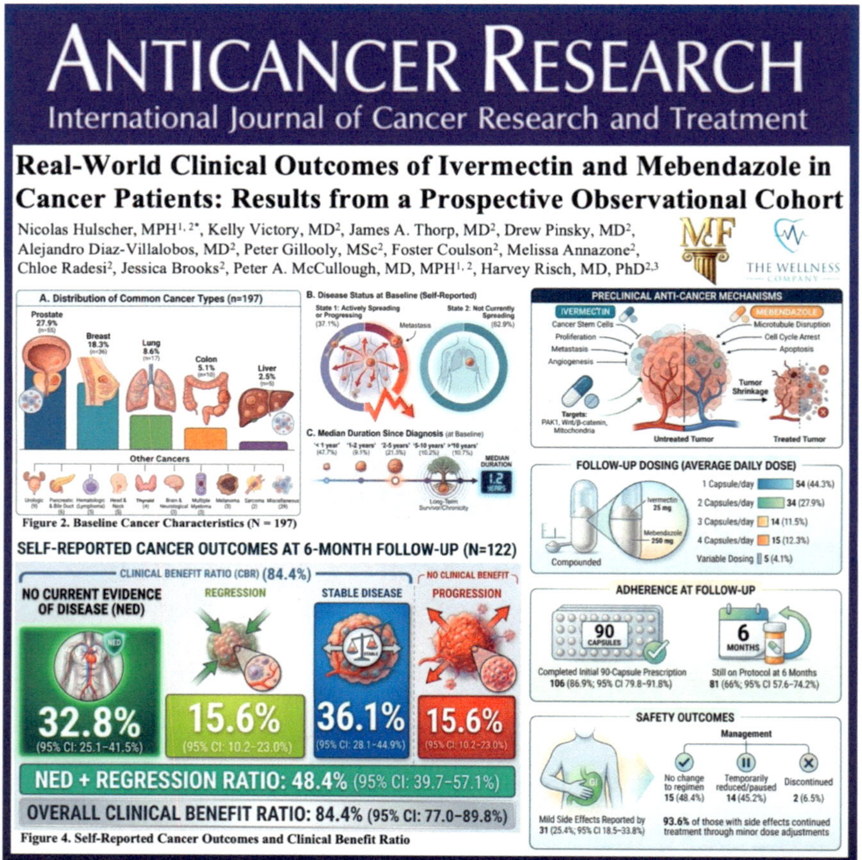

Real-World Clinical Outcomes of Ivermectin and Mebendazole in Cancer Patients: Results from a Prospective Observational Cohort:
Nicolas Hulscher, MPH, Kelly Victory, MD, James A. Thorp, MD, Drew Pinsky, MEF, Alejandro Diaz-Villalobos, MD2, Peter Gillooly, MSc, Foster Coulson, Melissa Annazone, Chloe Radesi, Jessica Brooks, Peter A. McCullough, MD, MPH, Harvey Risch, MD, PhD. PMID: 42203321.

June 2026 - Pubmed website: PMID 42203321

Parasites as cancer?

The theory that cancer is actually parasite activity is gaining traction, and seems to be borne out by the success of the anti-parasitic cancer protocols outlined by William Makis and others. As our surroundings, our air, water, food and our bodies have become more and more toxic, I believe we may have reduced the resilience we need to fend off parasitic infections which have been with us for a long time. This leaves us vulnerable to their multiplying and taking over.

For many years, the teeming world of parasites, from the microscopic intracellular parasites in our organs to the squirmy worms in our guts, has been largely ignored by western doctors. At the same time their veterinary colleagues were well aware that our pets and livestock needed regular attention to keep parasites at bay.

As seen in the clips on turbo cancers, where ordinary people are curing themselves with so called 'horse de-wormers' there appears to be a definite connection.

I went to the source for information on parasites and checked out Hulda Clark PhD (1928-2009) and 'The Cure for All Diseases'. This interesting book is compelling, although it must be admitted that Hulda herself died of cancer at the age of 80. For all that, she left a legacy which is still very valuable today.

She starts by telling us how to make her parasite 'zapper' ourselves. We can now buy them on Amazon ready to go. This simple frequency device was born out of the knowledge and research of Royal Raymond Rife, but is much more user friendly. With this device, you don't need to know exactly which parasites and frequencies you are zapping, the theory is that it covers many of them over about 20 minutes in a broad sweep.

Neither Royal Raymond Rife, or Hulda Clark patented their work, intending it to be freely available for everyone.

Having written this, I must add that the new nanotech contamination may not respond well to these frequency devices and care should be taken to check exactly what is happening in live blood if you use them.

Parasites are pesky little things too. They go through various stages in their life cycle and prefer to hide away in your cells, gut and tissues throughout them all. There might be generations of them tucked snugly out of sight in lumps and cysts waiting to cause problems. We have to use our wits to outsmart them.

It seems that parasites love toxic metals and I was interested to see a number of metals and parasites mentioned in Hulda's book which I had heard about before.

Elana Freeland and Maria Crisler have been talking about these same metals and parasites in connection with chemtrails: cadmium, aluminium, titanium strontium, and the particularly nasty parasite, ascaris, which Maria Crisler found in the artificial 'Florida Fog' which fell from the skies in 2025.

Hulda didn't like entertaining any of those parasites in any shape or form and recommended a scrupulously clean environment, including boiling underwear, covering soft furniture with plastic and getting rid of flowers, fitted carpets and pets. She wasn't keen on our furry friends, and saw them as carriers of parasites and disease.

This caution is emphasised by Dr Lee Merritt who never forgot being told during her training that one of the main risk factors for multiple sclerosis was having a dog in the house when you were a small child. Obviously small children crawl around on the floor with the pets and put all sorts of things into their mouths while they explore their world. Is multiple sclerosis actually caused by parasites?

While some of this seems quaint and extreme, Hulda has given us a legacy of a herbal parasite killing program which still forms the mainstay of many normal gut parasite cleanses today:

I have outlined it very briefly here but encourage you to look for it in full in her book, 'The Cure for All Diseases.'

Time for a reminder here that none of this is safe in pregnancy, especially as any parasite protocol is designed to hit the sweet spot between killing small organisms within our body without harming us. It's often a delicate balance. This is even more crucial in pregnancy when your growing baby is also a small organism in your body. All drugs, medicines, vaccines, alcohol and cigarettes should be avoided.

We all knew this sensible precaution when I had my children. It was just a couple of decades after mothers-to-be had been prescribed with Thalidomide for morning sickness in pregnancy. It had caused devastating injuries in at least 20,000 unborn babies world-wide. Doctors now gaily ignore warnings like this but they still stand the test of time. This is, sadly, more than we can say for many of today's procedures.

> Back in the day we ALL KNEW that you NEVER vaccinate a pregnant woman.
> No smoking, no alcohol, no vaccines and no medication (if humanly possible) if you want a healthy baby.
> We mums knew it.
> All the baby books knew it.
> The doctors and nurses knew it.
> Wise advice then.
> Wise advice now.

Herbal parasite killing program

Be guided by your gut, your intuition and your naturopath with this as a possible base suggestion.

Tincture of the green hull of the black walnut (extra strength) take one drop on an empty stomach in half a glass of filtered water.

Increase the dose drop-by-drop, day-by-day until day 6 when you are taking 2 teaspoons in a quarter glass of water.

Stop at day 6.

Wormwood capsules (I think there's a clue in the name here)
200-300 milligrams wormwood
Start with one capsule before dinner and increase day by day for two weeks until you are taking 7 capsules at once.
Stop at 17 days.

Ground Cloves (you can buy quality organic cloves to grind up fine in a spice grinder and put into empty capsules) or buy from a good source.
Start with 1 capsule, 3 times a day before meals
Increase over ten days until you are taking 3 capsules, 3 times a day.
Stop at 12 days

The maintenance program is:
One day per week:
Black wormwood tincture: 2 teaspoons before a meal in a little water.
Wormwood capsules: 7 taken together on an empty stomach.
Cloves: 3 capsules on an empty stomach.

Dr Ed Group and Global Healing Institute have a substantial paid course on removing parasites. As there is no doubt this process is not as simple as it seems, the course may be worth the investment if you want remove your own or guide others to do the same. The process will be made simpler by the fact that you can order the exact products needed from the Global Healing website.
https://globalhealing.com

There is a site recommended by Dr Lee Merritt: Cleanse Parasites which also has protocols and the exact ingredients needed to complete them.
https://cleanseparasites.com/

These processes seem to be so tailored, precisely timed and intricate that I think ordering the products you need from the company which has written the protocol makes a lot of sense.

Now What?

In the early days after the shock of seeing these filaments in my blood, I felt so alone in the midst of it, I sometimes felt as if it was all a bad dream. I didn't share it with many people because I didn't want to frighten them. The outside world still seemed so normal.

I found a number of people around the world who appear to be on similar journeys, notably the independent self-directed researchers like David Nixon's Micronauts. Most of them prefer to be anonymous and stay under the radar. Some, notably Dr Ana Milhacea, Dr David Nixon, Dr Ria Hayes, Maria Crisler and Dr Ed Group have bravely stepped up to raise the alarm.

This new contamination is strange and elusive. While unseen enemies in our skies are re-contaminating us nearly every day, I think getting rid of it all completely is optimistic. I believe it's a case of keeping it under control with constant action.

We still have far more questions than answers but after exploring this virgin bushland of strange and often conflicting information for many months, how far have we come?

We've been able to pick up a tiny handful of truths:

- This new contamination is real.
- It was hardly ever seen before 2021.
- It appears to self-assemble.
- It's very difficult to avoid.
- It affects nearly everyone.
- It's harmful to life.
- It can be deadly.
- It's being ignored by institutions.
- We need to rescue ourselves.
- We can get through this.

We've also picked up a tiny handful of clues:

There seems to be a wide and ever-changing variety of unwanted toxins being sprayed on us in chemtrails around the world.

The new contamination seems to be responsive to EMFs, frequency, temperature, oxygen levels, coherence, prayer and meditation.

It seems to appear in different forms in the blood: rogue fibrin and strange glowing lines and shapes lighting up our blood like fairy lights.

It seems that the delicate lining of the veins and arteries may be involved.

'We shall not cease from exploration, and the end of all our exploring will be to arrive where we started and know the place for the first time.'

T. S. Eliot

The Past

As we look to the future, we also have to truly acknowledge the past. We don't need to witness all the war crimes, but we do have to understand at least some of what has been done to millions of innocent, trusting people.

There is a time-honoured phrase we use to acknowledge their suffering. It's ironic that I am writing this during the eleventh hour of the eleventh day of the eleventh month 2025:

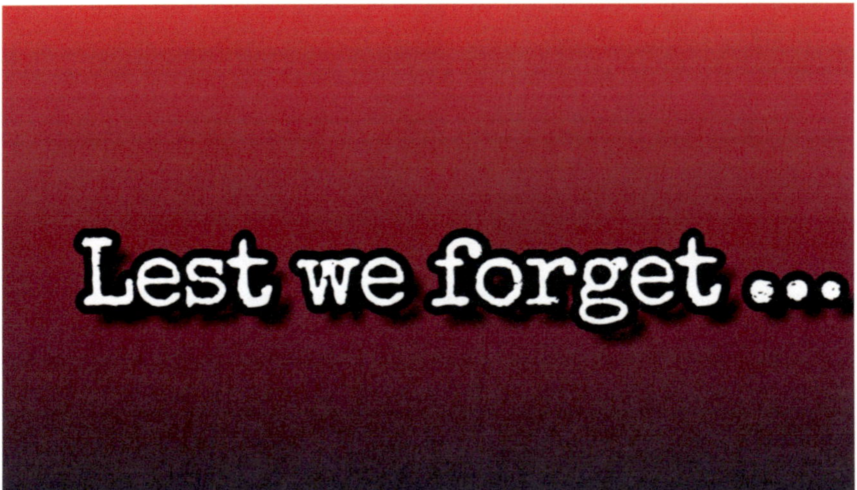

There is something very poignant and powerful about women and the vulnerable speaking uncomfortable truths. This is a perfect example as Dr Tess Lawrie reads the words of Margaret Anna Alice. Mistakes Were Not Made: An Anthem for Justice
https://youtu.be/ueUXNL-A3Zg

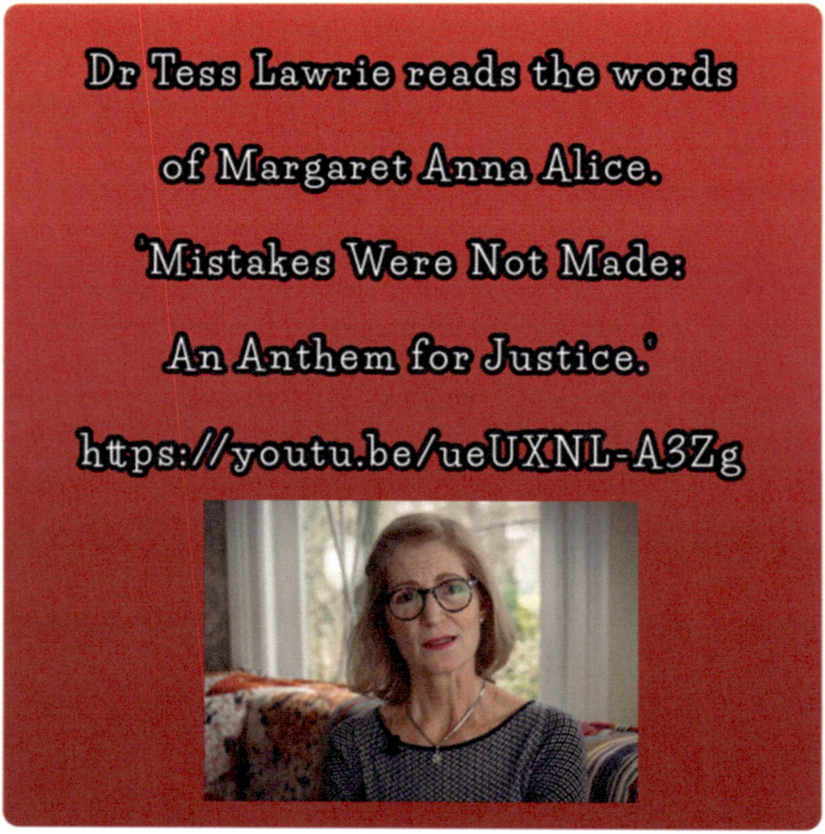

The Future

A first good, honest official response to any unnerving new blood contamination in the population would be that it is publicly acknowledged. As at July 2026, this is not yet happening. Many practitioners and clinics who are trying to heal people are not only being censored but threatened by the very institutions who should be supporting them. There is a reason why so many prefer to remain anonymous.

A second good, honest official response would be to stop the seemingly endless chemtrail and frequency contamination. Several states in the US have called for an end to them, so far without apparent success.

A third good, honest response would be to set egos and profits aside and pull together groups of university doctors, scientists and researchers to work together with independent microscopists to share ideas and resources, so we can learn how to restore our health more quickly.

A fourth good, honest response would be to fund and issue therapeutic packs to help people to clear their blood.

So far, the vast wealth and resources of our universities, medical schools and research facilities has not been used to even look at, let alone study this subject.

In a compartmentalised world, it's easy for these institutions to pretend that the projects they are working on are for the benefit of humanity. Are they really?

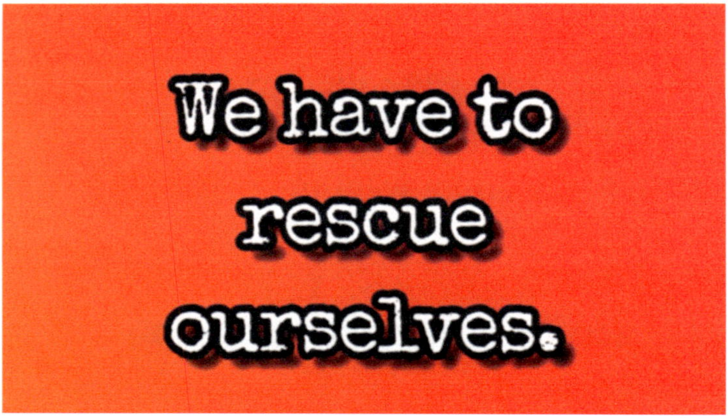

We need the people who are tracking down and interpreting who is responsible for chemtrails and other poisons in our skies.

We need the intrepid teams of independent Micronauts around the world to interpret the nuances of whatever is happening in our blood, sweat and tears.

We need the technology and practitioners who are physically able to filter our blood and pull out the rubbery clots before it's too late.

We need the people who are spreading the word about how we can start to clear these contaminants out of our blood with supplements, lasers and other means.

NO GUARANTEES

We might think about our new task as a new fitness routine. As individuals, we need to pick up our health and fitness game, head to the gym and clean up the diet. We may need to do the colon cleanses and liver cleanses. We may need to check our nutrient levels and invest in organic foods and natural supplements to escape the poisoning as best we can. We need to find good, open-minded naturopaths and other practitioners to help us. I have put together some suggestions as best I can in this book. We might choose one from the list that feels right and give it a go. Maybe cycle it with another one in whatever way works for us. We need to believe that all will be well.

If we're lucky, we'll be able to track down a live blood analysis practitioner and check our progress.

Most of all, we need to hold the faith. We need to maintain the faith in ourselves and in our bodies that we can overcome this.

We are far more powerful and resilient than we've been led to believe. We, the people, have overcome plagues, wars, famines, genocides, mind control, concentration camps, exile, blood sacrifice, satanic ritual abuse, shootings, bombings, slavery, poisoning, floods, fires, snow storms and hurricanes - and we're still here.

I'll leave the closing words to the ever prophetic and insightful Alex Collier, who has offered us consistent, measured insight and wisdom from his unique perspective for over 30 years.

'The people as a whole have more common sense than all the governments in the world. We always figure it out.'

Alex Collier
Andromedan contactee

Websites

Global Healing

globalhealing.com
globalhealinginstitute.org

Dr Edward Group's company, Global Healing is at the leading edge of finding solutions for the nanotech which is contaminating us. The company is constantly looking for better ways of supporting the body to rid itself of it.

Dr Group has had a huge wealth of experience in teams studying the effectiveness of many healing modalities over the years.

His supplement company prides itself being rigorous about quality, testing both initial samples and bulk deliveries on a regular basis. Their exceptional quality can be seen in special photography which captures their auras.

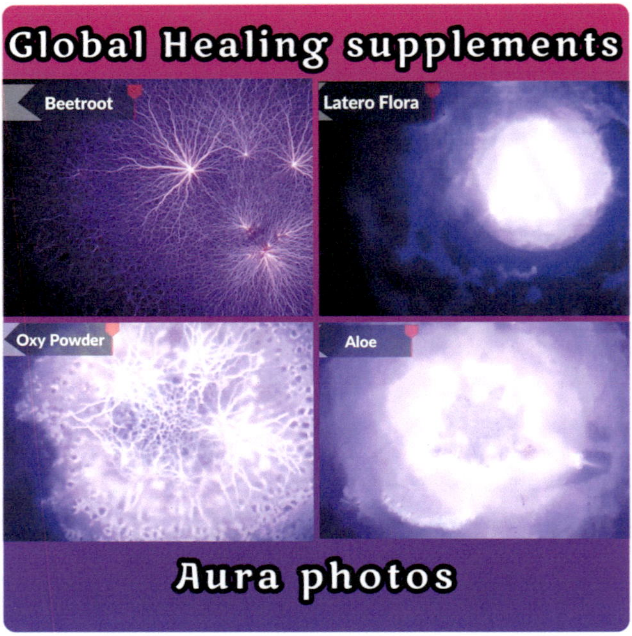

Global Healing also has many educational videos and you can even invest in their certified health coach training program. I think this might be a great option for people who would like to learn to help others recover from this toxic world.

Dr Group appears to be one of the inner-circle advising Secretary of Health and Human Services Robert F Kennedy Jr, which I find reassuring.

Dr Group and Global Healing are on the front line addressing the nanofilament issue.

The Dr Ardis Show

Thedrardisshow.com

I really struggled with Bryan's flamboyant style when he first appeared on shows talking about snake venoms. It all seemed a bit wild and over the top.

There's a back story to that style which makes so much sense. Bryan Ardis was the eldest child of five in a family who moved interstate frequently to follow their father's career.

He constantly questioned the world around him and felt that it was his responsibility to look after his younger siblings and teach them about the ways of the world.

I can picture him as a boy with his wavy hair, dressed in his shorts and T-shirt with his little brothers and sisters gathered around him, hanging on his every word. I fancy a bit of that inquisitive, well intentioned and dramatic teacher has stayed with him.

Since he first arrived on the scene in 2021, He has brought incredible insights to the covid plandemic, backed with ample research. Dr Bryan Ardis is a retired chiropractor. In Australia we are used to chiropractors not involving themselves in the world of prescription drugs, hospitals or even supplements, but in the US, their area of study and expertise is much broader, encompassing pharmacy and even (like Dr Sherri Tenpenny) emergency medicine.

As he writes in his book, 'Moving Beyond the Covid 19 Lies' he was drawn into the covid situation after witnessing the gruelling and completely unnecessary death of his father-in-law in hospital. This experience alerted him to other anomalies in hospital procedures and he made the decision to go public with what he knew about the dangers of Remdesivir. It was a hint from another doctor who alerted him to the snake venom industry. His dedicated research first unearthed two types of snake venom which had been used in many batches, and then he discovered that a total of 36 manufactured snake and snail venoms had been carefully collected from around the world and used in various formulations.

He was well aware of the danger he and his family faced from the pharmaceutical industry by revealing this information.

If you are suffering after covid shots, chapter 15 of his book contains a number of medical tests and the natural protocols to remedy them. This is a very valuable resource which I won't replicate here, but at

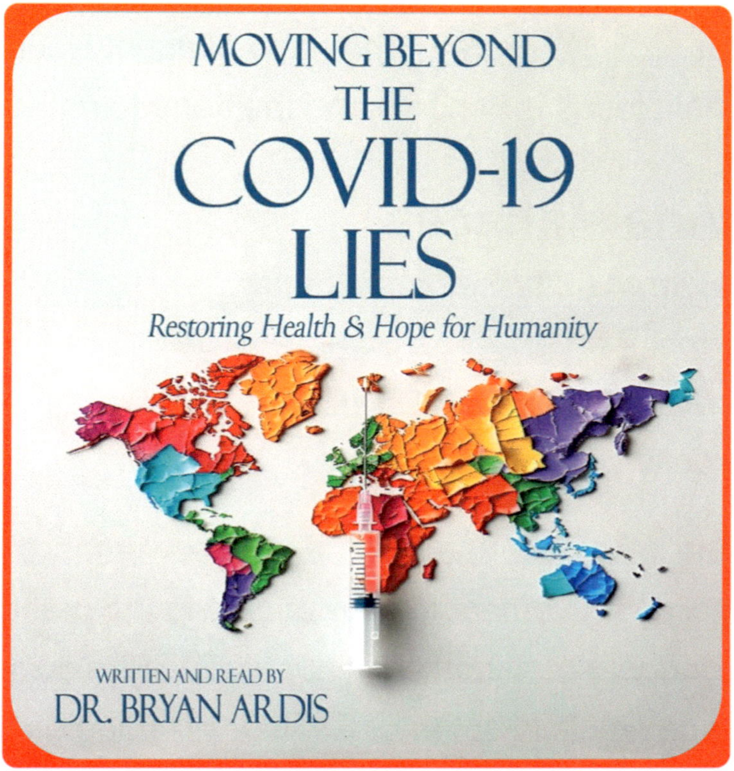

least you know where to find it.

Brian is also known as the Nicotine guy, and has been a major voice for truth in the post-covid era. You can buy a number of relevant supplements and listen to interviews with interesting specialists on his website. As he is a close friend and colleague of Dr Ed Group, I would guess that his supplements would be of a high quality.

Bryan Ardis is aware of the nano-filament issue but his main focus is venoms and their antidotes.

Dr Ana Milhacea

https://dranamihalcea.com/about

Substacks

Ana Maria Milhacea MD PhD

Humanity United Now

Dr Ana Milhacea has been a spokeswoman of the fledgeling movement to alert people to the presence and dangers of nanotech in our blood. She owns an anti-ageing clinic south of Seattle, Washington, and was doing live blood analysis, EDTA and other blood cleansing therapies at the clinic when she started to find the nanotech in people's blood in late 2021. These fluorescent particles had seldom been seen before then.

She has written three books:

Light Medicine - a new Paradigm - the Science of Light, Spirit and Longevity.

Transhuman - Volume 1. The Real Covid 19 Agenda.

Transhuman – Volume 2. Overcoming the Global Depopulation Agenda.

She has given many interviews on this subject and has been very outspoken. Not everyone agrees with all her conclusions.

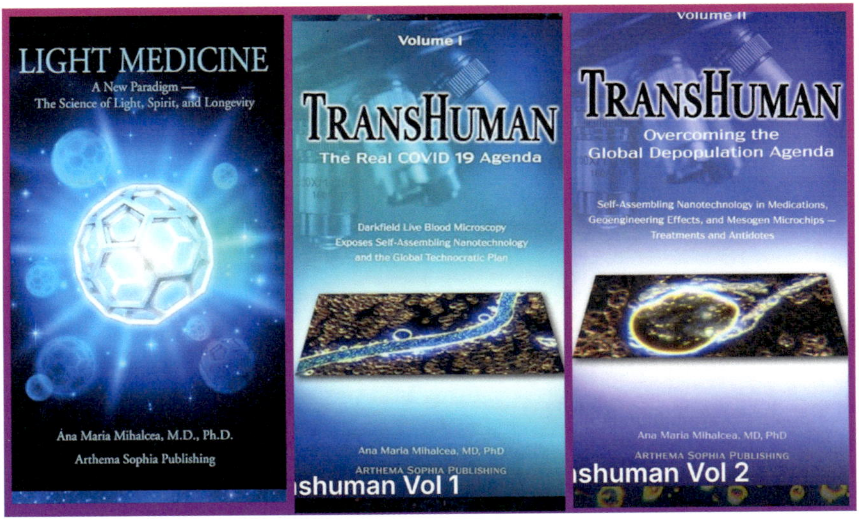

Her last book does include some very relevant solutions but her focus in many of her talks and books has been warning about the problem. Once we understand the problems, I believe it's more important for doctors and scientists to focus on how we get this artificial contamination out of us.

Ana Milhacea's posts and interviews on nanotech in the blood can be found on Substack, Rumble and elsewhere.

Evolving Solutions

www.evolvingsolutions.world

www.longhaulers.world

nomoreslience - Rumble channel

This organisation is one of those at the heart of helping people this situation both on line and in clinic. There are now a number of Evolve clinics in the UK, Palma and Cyprus which routinely conduct physical EBOO, EDTA and other related treatments for those suffering with long covid and other symptoms. People visit these clinics from around the world and the team frequently pull rubbery clots and 'coffee grounds' clots out of the veins and arteries.

Dr Ria Hayes has been an amazing source of insight on this issue to me and the Evolving Solutions Membership Portal will make trusted information much easier to access. This team works in collaboration with Dr Ed Group of Global Healing, Bryan Ardis and Maria Crisler of Abeytu Naturals. Their main focus is to spread awareness of a range of remedies and treatments.

Join the Evolving Solutions Membership Portal for a very small fee.
I find gentle English voices very reassuring.

Abeytu Naturals

abeytunaturals.com
mariacrisler.com

Maria Crisler is an expert in clinical microbiology and hematology (the study of blood.) Her focus is exploring how modern technology, the environment and synthetic chemicals and toxins impact human biology.

She works in collaboration with Global Healing and others and has also developed a few of her own award-winning therapeutic products under the Abeytu Naturals brand.

Maria is one of the handful of people in the world who analyses the contents of chemtrails, 'Florida fog', unusual snow, nano-micro filaments and other chemicals to assess the danger to human beings.

Maria's main focus is on chemtrails and remedies for nanotech and other contaminants in the blood.

Carnicom Institute

https://carnicominstitute.org/
Carnicom Institute Substack

For nearly 30 years, independent scientist Clifford Carnicom has been researching how chemtrails and wireless 5G/6G electromagnetics are essential to geoengineering and bioengineering. His website of 450 papers and photographs guides viewers through decades of research to the present day merging of what is coming from the sky and Big Pharma's global inoculations.

Elana Freeland

Elana is one of the original meticulous researchers of the transhuman agenda, keeping a watchful eye on government, regulation, HAARP, chemtrails and nanotechnology in the US. She has written five books about geoengineering, spelling out how geoengineering interfaces with synthetic biology and present-day chronic illnesses. You can buy these on Amazon or listen to them on Audiobooks. Her most recent book is The Geoengineered Transhuman (2025) and she is now working on a book with independent scientist Clifford Carnicom.

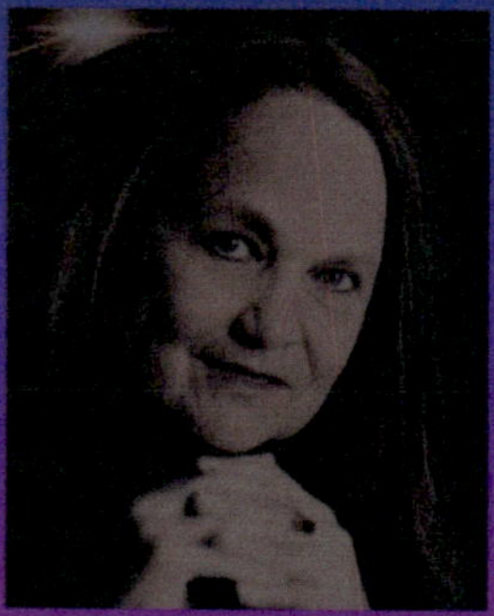

Elana Freeland MA: books
THE GEOENGINEERING TRILOGY:
Geoengineered Transhumanism: How the Environment Has Been Weaponized by Chemicals, Electromagnetism & Nanotechnology for Synthetic Biology (2021)
Under An Ionized Sky: From Chemtrails to Space Fence Lockdown (2018)
Chemtrails, HAARP, and the Full Spectrum Dominance of Planet Earth (2014)

Dr David Nixon

drdavidnixon.com

www.thegreatbritishbookshop.co.uk

Dr David B Nixon was a General Practitioner for over 25 years and was suspended in late 2023 for writing exemptions from the covid shots in line with the Nuremberg Code.

He bought a dark field microscope in 2022 to study the shots and the blood of curious friends. He's created a variety of publications to record, publicise and attempt to understand these unusual new anomalies.

The Nixonlab Soft Matter Library:

The Atlas of Soft Matter Structures

The Atlas of Soft Matter Structures in Blood.

Soft Matter in Motion

The Quiet work of Health

Playing with Pfire

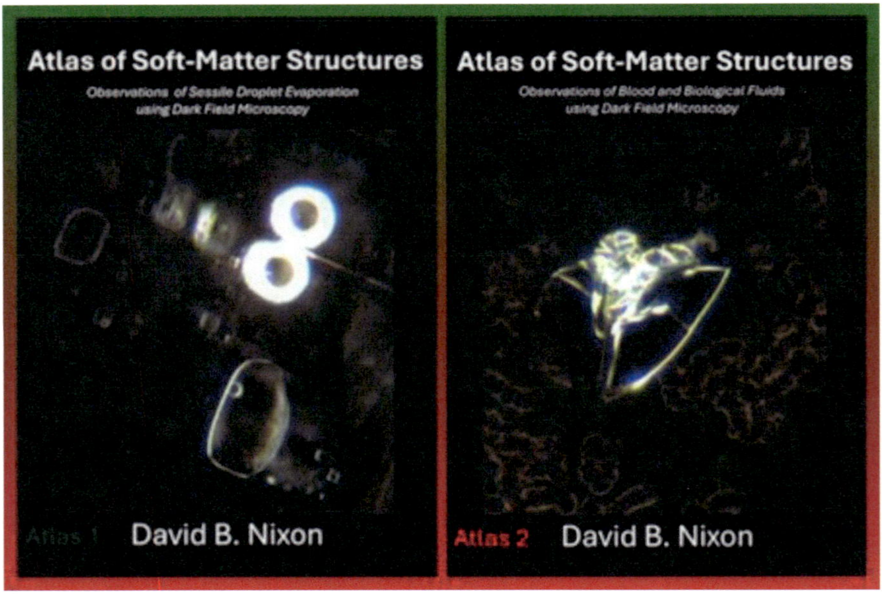

The Micronauts

The Micronauts are an informal international group of independent microscopists, clinicians, researchers, and observers facilitated by Dr David Nixon. Since 2023, the group has met online to share self-directed investigations using optical microscopy, with particular attention to blood, biological fluids, environmental samples, pharmaceutical preparations and other materials of interest.

The group provides a forum for observation, discussion, technical exchange, comparison of findings, and critical debate. Over time, its work has increasingly been informed by a soft-matter perspective, with attention to fields, boundaries, gels, fibres, vesicular domains, crystalline structures, phase behaviour, and time-dependent organisation in complex fluids and drying preparations.

Members come from varied backgrounds, including human and veterinary medicine, dentistry, chemistry, environmental science, live blood analysis, photography, computing, engineering, and independent research. Each participant remains responsible for their own observations, interpretations, publications, and public statements. The Micronauts are not a formal institution, professional body, or funded research organisation.

Geoengineering Watch

geoengineeringwatch.org

Dane Wigington

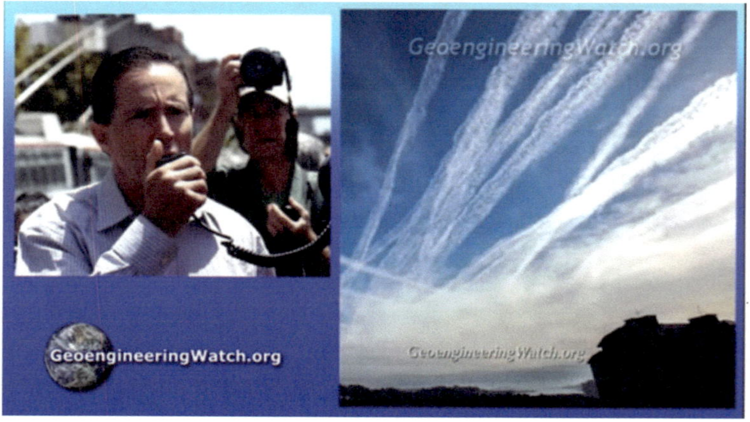

Dane has devoted the last 20 years of his life to research into secret global climate and geoengineering operations and the effort to expose and halt them. He is scientific and precise in his communication He was the executive producer on the documentary 'The Dimming' which you can find on the website.

He is one of the world authorities in this field.

Biglesen Academy

https://bigelsenacademy.com/

Harvey Bigleson 1940-2019

It is important to note that the founder of this family business died at the age of 79, the year before the covid plandemic started. He linked the state of the blood to emotions and spoke of anomalies in the blood as holograms.

Who knows what he would have made of the situation we face now?

His sons, operating under the name of The Bigelsen Academy, work mainly with blood samples people have taken themselves and mailed in. (Having noted the great care with which my naturopath collects the finger-prick blood properly and tests it immediately, before it degrades, this seems unusual.) They make no comment about the vast increase in blood anomalies we are seeing since 2022 and claim that the filaments are holographic and nothing new.

This opinion is not borne out by any of the experienced live blood analysis people I have encountered, many of whom have been working with blood analysis for over a decade. This includes my first shocking encounter in the naturopath's office witnessing these filaments in my own blood.

In my opinion, we ignore the reality of nano-micro filaments in our blood and their relation to rubbery clots at our peril.

The Wellness Company (USA)

https://www.twc.health

This company still has its line-up of courageous and outspoken doctors, tele-health practitioners, useful supplements and medications. Prices are not exactly cheap and medication is still very much part of the treatments on offer, but I think you are more likely to encounter a practitioner who will work with you in good conscience for your benefit than you are in completely mainstream health companies.

They are not addressing the nano-tech issue publicly as at early 2026.

Dr Lee Merrit

Dr. Lee Merritt
The Medical Rebel

drleemerritt.com

Rumble Channel: The Medical Rebel

I really like Dr Lee Merritt, a former orthopaedic surgeon from a medical family. She has years of experience in the medical business, a sense of humour and a wonderful ability to think outside the box. She has some very interesting articles, videos and interviews on her website, where you can also find a small collection of health and detox products.

She believes that most cancers are caused by parasites and has a very interesting parasite cleanse video and protocol available on her website.
Lee Merritt is aware of the nano-filaments.

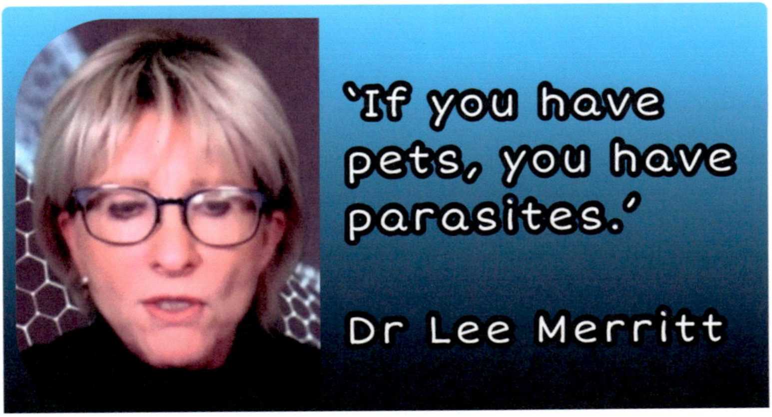

ELFET/Tri-Vortex

This company brings to market a unique and revolutionary range of products, which have benefit for many biological systems.

It has been discovered that their green laser technology, which will fit into your pocket, is very beneficial for helping the body clear nano-micro tech.

www.elfet.org

sales@elfet.org

In Australia, contact:

rob@everleaf.com.au

Helix Institute

56 Barry's Point Road, Takapuna,
Auckland 0622

health@helixinstitute.nz

A beautiful new holistic health hub. One of the very few clinics in the Southern hemisphere offering EBOO, and Weber green laser therapies.

Kirsty Bednar ND, BHSc (Comp Med) EmpowerU Natural Health

Elder Street, Lambton
Newcastle NSW
https://www.kirstybednar.com/

Kirsty Bednar is an inspiration on this journey. She has been a naturopath and live blood analysis specialist for 20 years and empowers her clients to take control of their health and well-being. She uses a holistic approach that addresses the mind, body, and spirit. guiding them towards a happier and healthier life

Independent Medical Alliance

imahealth.org

This organisation used to be known as the FLCCC (Front Line Critical Covid Care). It was founded by Dr Paul Marik and Dr Pierre Kory, two doctors at the top of their field who had lost jobs for standing up against the mandated covid shots.

The aim is to discuss and practice honest medicine. This sets it apart from the mainstream medical business and there is a wealth of knowledge and clues on here on how to get to the heart of symptoms in the post covid era. Clients in the US can find a list of open-minded professionals on their website.

As at May 2026, they don't appear to address the new contamination issue.

World Council for Health

worldcouncilforhealth.com

The World Council for Health is an international association which offers a wealth of unbiased holistic, medical and general wellbeing advice. It is free from the shackles of vested interests.

It has united 230 like-minded organisations spanning 55 countries and representing honest, health focussed voices around the world and empowered by science and wisdom.

There are various protocols and areas of study that you can access for a small fee.

Although they do include a spike detox protocol on their website, at this stage they don't appear to be addressing the new contamination issue specifically.

World of Wellness

https://wowintl.org

World of Wellness is an Australian organisation led by the courageous and tireless Professor Ian Brighthope. It unites many ethical practitioners in holistic medicine, health, insurance and law to offer wise advice and counsel to any politicians and government agencies who care to listen.

It offers members trusted health advice and a curated list of wholistic and independent practitioners.

Dr Joe Dispenza

https://drjoedispenza.com

Dr Joe Dispenza's groundbreaking and verified work spans the divide between the power of the mind, body, heart and soul to restore and heal.

Mind Movies

mindmovies.com

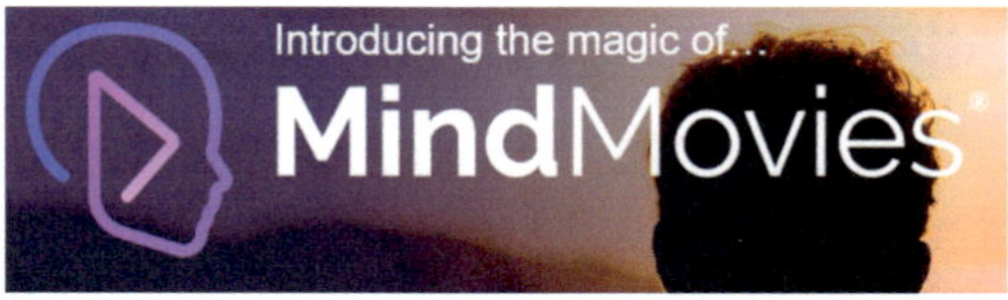

For a fee, this website allows you to make your own advert for the life (and the health) you want.

Have fun and design your future....

McCullough Foundation

https://mcculloughfnd.org/

Dr Peter McCullough found out how quickly the US medical industry turns on you when you start to question their narrative. In 2022 he was shocked to find himself being pushed from the very top of his field and thrown out on his ear within months.

Since then, he has spoken out courageously, shining light on many studies which the medical industry would prefer to keep hidden in the shadows.

'When fear is weaponized against the people, truth is the only defence.'

At this stage the foundation has not publicly addressed the new contamination we face.

Live Blood Analysis Training

I hope that my efforts with this book may have encouraged a few people, especially naturopaths, to take a closer look at incorporating live blood analysis into their clinics. Here are what appear to be the best websites offering both certified training and specials on the most appropriate microscopes. All training can be done on-line and at long distance.

Naturecure Academy

www.livebloodanalysistraining.com/

I like the clear way the Naturecure Academy presents its certified courses and the specials for appropriate dark field microscopes and monitor-linked cameras.

Naturecure
ACADEMY

WELCOME TO THE CENTRE OF EXCELLENCE FOR STUDENTS FROM AROUND THE WORLD

I have been told that the microscopes available through this company are of a good quality. Most of the courses are on line

Live Blood Online

https://livebloodonline.com/

This course is led by Dr Okker Botha, a homeopathic doctor with many years' experience. It is one of the most in-depth online courses available. I have been told that the online course was excellent and even more useful as it can be repeated many times while you learn. This course also includes guidance on the choice of a dark field microscope and linked camera set up.

With this new contamination I believe we need all the live blood analysts we can get, possibly working alongside naturopaths and other holistic practitioners. I hope this offers some inspiration.

Don't Look Away

Don't look away
because what you see
makes you feel uncomfortable.
Let curiosity be your guide
and truth your destination.

For every mistake made for not doing
ten are made for not looking.
Let's make less miss takes.

What use is the spotlight
revealing the truth
when nobody's looking?

'Tis the tree falling in the forest
Without a sound
Without a witness.

– David B. Nixon 2026

Thank You

Stacey P. Nadine S. Lee C.
David Nixon. Tobias Beharrell.
Alyce. Larry. Sam. Matt. Shelley.
Iain. Rob Caruso. Fiona.
Sparkles. Kirsty Bednar.
Angie Starbright. Karen B. Elise.
Megan. Carole.
Freedom Warrior W.
The Micronauts. Ana Milhacea,
Ria Hayes. Ed Group.
Maria Crisler. Karen Wilds.

Links and References

Some of the information in this enormous line up may be disturbing to some people. I've included some of it to give people starter points for further investigation which may help us put a stop to this. If you are reading this book to rescue yourself, you may like to stay on the healing side of it all rather than attempt to unpick the depressing details of where it's coming from.

Suppliers

Miracle Products

https://miracleproducts.shop/

Manufacturer and supplier of a range of high quality supplements and therapeutics in Australia.

They include Blu-Zone methylene blue, CDS tabs for water purification, DMSO, and Nascent Iodine. There is a lot of information about these products on their website.

Metagenics

Metagenics.com.au

Highly regarded brand of supplements and therapeutics usually supplied through a naturopath.

Garden of Life

Gardenoflife.com

I really like this range of quality, herb-based supplements (Even though they have been bought out by a pharma company) They are now available in Australia through iHerb.

iHerb

https://au.iherb.com

This well-known supplier carries a huge range of different supplement and health brands. We need to do our own research to check the quality of the particular band we are considering.

Richardson Nutritional Center

Following in the footsteps of Dr John Richardson, a B17 pioneer

https://rncstore.com/

: est On Earth products

bestonearthproducts.com

A wide range of products including black salve

Advanced Tachyon Technologies

https://store.planet-tachyon.com/#

Tachyon EMF protection products as recommended by Dr Gabriel Cousens:

ELFET/Tri-Vortex information

Tri-Vortex green laser, Tri-Vortex chamber, Tri-Vortex treated water-structuring discs

www.elfet.org

Yoodok

Weber green laser

https://www.yoodok.health/about-yoodok

Orgonite Pyramids (in Australia)

Email: jasminebalconi@outlook.com

All Natural Deodorant.

Despite the limited scope of the name, this Australian website offers a lot of useful information and therapeutics

https://allnaturaldeodorant.com.au

Extension Health

If you happen to be in New York, you are fully catered for by this young team in these amazing clinics.

https://extension.health/services

: ooks

Wendy Daniel

(I get pride of place for my own books in this line up)

Links and references for all three books are live on my website

https://www.lightoftruths.net/

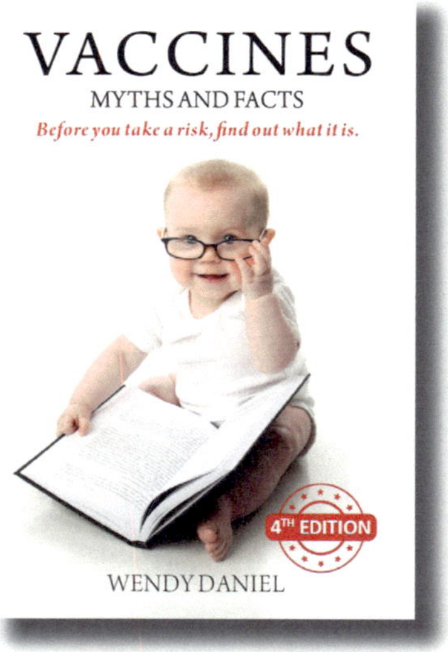

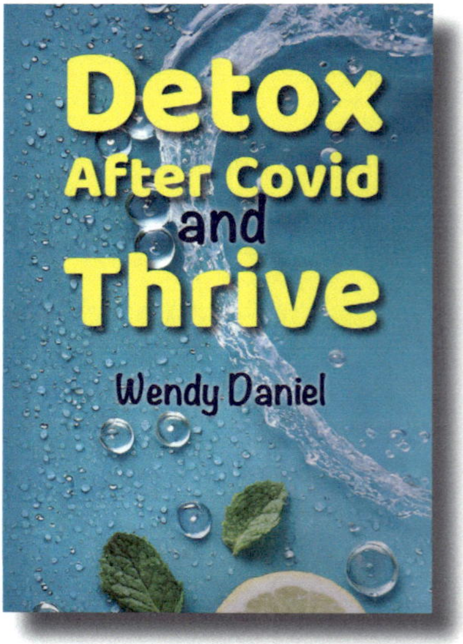

Vaccines, Myths and Facts, (4th Edition 2023)

Now on Amazon Kindle. Big text, lots of pics and graphs, so easy to read a ten-year-old can understand it and 100 links and references (often to original studies) on the website

https://www.lightoftruths.net/

It's something of a portal to the avalanche of information that mainstream is still trying to hide... Get the physical book from: *www.inhousebookstore.com.au*

A talk about the 4th edition of 'Vaccines, Myths and Facts': *https://youtu.be/SfS03lYAZIQ?si=Ai3tJrljaHTroT_J.*

Detox after Covid and Thrive, (2024)

This book is a great start to the post covid detox journey for newcomers. It takes you from being mainstream medicine compliant to navigating your own journey to health. Some simple things you can do yourself, some supplements you may have heard about, how and when to choose a good practitioner, nine websites at the leading edge of covid recovery and TEN successful case histories from Australian naturopaths.

https://www.lightoftruths.net/

It's on Amazon Kindle or in hard copy from *www.inhousebookstore.com.au*

A talk about 'Detox after Covid and Thrive' *https://youtu.be/MsN_8stSv3Y?si=svJG7b3C3-GD7HlX*

Anna Milhacea:

Light Medicine: The science of light, spirit and longevity

Transhuman – the real covid 19 agenda

Transhumanism – Overcoming the global depopulation agenda.

'The work compiled in this book is my contribution for the survival of our species and the future of humanity' Dr Ana Milhacea. 17 August 2024.

Elana Freeland:

A prolific writer about the detailed back stories and origins of Geoengineering.

Chemtrails, HAARP, and the Full Spectrum Dominance of Planet Earth (2014)

Under an Ionized Sky: From Chemtrails to Space Fence Lockdown (2018)

Geoengineered Transhumanism: How the Environment Has Been Weaponized by Chemicals, Electromagnetics, & Nanotechnology for Synthetic Biology (2021)

The Sub Rosa America series (a multi-volume work of fictionalized deep political history)

: ryan Ardis:

Moving Away from Covid 19 Lies.

An outspoken chiropractor's journey through the recent deception and how to protect yourself from it.

Dr David : Nixon

The Atlas of Soft Matter Structures: Observations from Dark Field Microscopy and Sessile Droplet Evaporation.

The Atlas of Soft Matter Structures in Blood: The ebb and flow of bodily fluids, membranes, structures and functions

Soft Matter in Motion:

The Quiet work of Health: Principles for self-management in a new health era.

Playing with Pfire: This is the first volume of a series of visual and poetic reflections – fragments of a world in transition - without filters or fabrication.

David Nixon was a Brisbane based general practitioner for 25 years. His subsequent dark field microscopy work is important to anyone wishing to understand the detail of this new contamination.

drdavidnixon.com

: arbara O'Neill

https://officialbarbaraoneill.com

https://www.mmh.com.au

Self Heal by Design

Sustain Me.

These are a wealth of basic common sense and natural healing information.

Dr Pierre Kory

The War on Ivermectin.

A doctor negotiates the covid plandemic era.

Robert F Kennedy Jr

The Real Anthony Fauci: Bill Gates, Big Pharma, and the Global War on Democracy and Public Health (2021)

For many years I have found Robert F Kennedy Jr to be very thoroughly researched and accurate.

Aaron Siri:

Vaccines, Amen. The lawyer dismantling the corrupt practices so endemic in the vaccine industry, one FOI request, deposition and court case at a time.

Unhackable Publications

NANO NANO: Microscopy Investigations

A collection of over 300 colour microscopy images showcased from an international group of independent microscopists known as the Micronauts. The book reveals hundreds of examples of assembled synthetic biology and nanotechnology contaminating our bodies and our environment.

Substack: Free@Un-Hackable Animal

Tobias :eharrell

Breath of Fresh Air:

A book about nebulizing.

Eileen McKusick:

Tuning the Human Biofield.

Electric Body, Electric Health.

I have listened to Eileen's books several times. They are scientific, practical, thorough and easy to understand. I believe they are important as a background to this aspect of our being.

Peter A Kirby

Chemtrails Exposed. More in depth information

Dr Steven A Ross PhD

Shattered. My personal experiences with the Universal Microscope. The story of Royal Raymond Rife and his life-giving inventions.

More on-line resources

The HighWire. Rumble

Del Bigtree

This organisation, together with its related organisation, ICAN (Informed Consent Action Network) has created a

strong foundation of information and powerful legal action challenging the vaccine narrative. They turned their attention to the geoengineering issue in early 2026.
https://rumble.com/c/TheHighWire

Dr Eric Berg. YouTube

Clear, simple information about almost any medical information you can think of.
This doctor has censored himself enough to keep his YouTube channel but gives consistent, excellent, balanced insights within those boundaries.
https://youtube.com/@drberg?si=86sGdkGIcsHnQvws

Dr John Campbell. YouTube

Initially a believer in the covid situation, Dr John Campbell followed the real science wherever it went, translating medical and scientific research into simple language we can all understand. Although he has censored himself enough to keep his YouTube channel, he made a complete turnaround early on in the plandemic and has brought many followers with him to continue questioning everything.

Ria No More Silence: Facebook

Nomoresilence: Rumble

Detailed information and clips of what is going on in the blood.

'The Truth about Cancer'

Ty and Charlene Bollinger.

A great resource: YouTube, Rumble

https://thetruthaboutcancer.com/

'Cancer Decoded'

A wonderful resource by Jonathon Otto and dozens of knowledgeable guest speakers.

https://www.youtube.com › watch?v=BW6SlvIxzKg

Tobias Beharrell Tobias Lab

https://www.tobiaslab.com/training

Tobias is a wealth of professional information for professionals Tobias is acutely aware of the new contamination and natural ways to keep it under control.

Systems Regulation in Clinical Practice

Advanced practitioner training in clinical decision architecture and physiological signal interpretation for complex physiological cases.

Margaret Anna Alice

Mistakes were not made.

An Anthem for Justice

Read by Dr Tess Lawrie

https://youtu.be/ueUXNL-A3Zg

As at June 2026, all these links were live and all can be found on my website: https://www.lightoftruths.net/

Watch out for pesky little gaps that appear in the links stopping them working. I found Google by far the best search engine for this. Copy the link and paste it into Google. Three copies of the link will come up. Use one that isn't live and check it very carefully for gaps There may be a couple of them on longer links. Closing them up on the link that wasn't live will correct them on the live link so you can go straight to the piece.

I don't necessarily agree with all the information, but I do believe it's important to our exploration.

Origins of the onslaught

Nanotech Patents

https://open.substack.com/pub/eccentrik/p/we-just-hit-the-motherload?r=149bj4&utm_medium=ios

Chemtrails, the suppliers' trade association

https://x.com/bgatesisapyscho/status/2029271539980415330?s=46&t=nkWTOBihgJ1KldA6v7wgHQ

The History of Nanoscience and Nanotechnology: From Chemical-Physical Applications to Nanomedicine

Nanoscience is a convergence of physics, materials science and biology, which deal with manipulation of materials at atomic and molecular scales; while nanotechnology is the ability to observe measure, manipulate, assemble, control, and manufacture matter at the nanometer scale. 2019

https://pmc.ncbi.nlm.nih.gov/articles/PMC6982820/

PMID: 31892180.

How did we get where we are today? The transhumanism agenda explained by Ed Group of Global Healing

What we're really looking at is a system capable of engineering droughts, floods and storms, shifting climates, and rewriting natural weather patterns, all in plain sight.

https://rumble.com/v5jdwzp-how-did-we-get-where-we-are-today-transhumanism-agenda-explained.html

5G and the Wireless Body Area Network

Sabrina Wallace is the hard edge of this discussion and may be the one who is closest to the truth. Seemorerocks

https://open.substack.com/pub/seemorerocks/p/sabrina-wallace-they-are-truning?r=149bj4&utm_medium=ios

Why are human bodies emitting a signal from beyond the grave?

https://youtu.be/GSJ2GHI_AdM?si=VPviUkiNMVn3-IJC

Dr Ed Group talks about strontium, cesium and other elements in the nano-filaments and chemtrails

https://www.facebook.com/share/r/19AbYTG9bz/?mibextid=wwXIfr

More chemtrail ingredients

https://x.com/iluminatibot/status/2030893901553315901?s=

Dane Wigington of Geoengineering Watch talks about chemtrails to Tucker Carlson.

https://x.com/iluminatibot/status/2023178054198247681?s=46&t=nkWTOBihgJ1KldA6v7wgHQ

Man in America talks to Kim Bright about chemtrails.
The frightening truth about weather warfare and depopulation.

https://rumble.com/v6w7svo-the-frightening-truth-about-weather-warfare-and-depopulation-w-kim-bright.html

Karen Kingston reports on patents held by the pharmaceutical company Moderna

https://rumble.com/v5yqkaz-karen-kingston-reports-on-patents-held-by-the-pharmaceutical-company-modern.html

A pilot speaks about the covid shots and their impact:
https://www.instagram.com/reel/DOL_TsiCbTy/?igsh=MWhza3k2ZG1tcXRiZg==

Clifford Carnicon from the Carnicon Institute talks about his 25 years of laboratory work on Chemtrails
https://audio.solari.com/sr20240702/sr20240702_Interview.mp3

Robert F Kennedy Jr Interviews Kris Newby author of 'Bitten', The terrible, truly awful back story of Bioweapons & Lyme Disease
https://rumble.com/v48ge19-rfk-jr.-interviews-kris-newby-the-terrible-truly-awful-backstory-of-bioweap.html

The origin of Lyme disease?
https://x.com/red_pill_us/status/1951785698438345140?s=46&t=nkWTOBihgJ1KldA6v7wgHQ

Declassified Documents Link U.S.Bioweapons Program to Lyme Disease Outbreak
https://www.malone.news/p/declassified-documents-link-us-bioweapons

Lyme disease naturopath
https://x.com/skriptkeeper17/status/2040795877598486601?s=46&t=nkWTOBihgJ1KldA6v7wgHQ

BITTEN: How Ticks Are Turning Meat-Eaters Into Allergy Victims
The HighWire has a few shows on ticks and lyme disease.
https://rumble.com/v7aa5ak-ticks-alpha-gal.html

Cross Domain Bacteria, AKA Morgellons
https://open.substack.com/pub/woodnstone820/p/cross-domain-bacteria-aka-morgellons?r=149bj4&utm_medium=ios

Space Fence & Mind Control
A Conversation with Elana Freeland.
Truth, Science and Spirit Ep 52
Ana Milhacea talks to Elana Freeland
https://anamihalceamdphd.substack.com/p/space-fence-and-mind-control-conversation?r=149bj4&utm_medium=ios&utm_campaign=audio-player

This section is a deep rabbit hole about the development of some of this technology. It is not for the faint hearted in either content or delivery.

If you Google Sabrina Wallace quite a lot of information will come up from her interesting background and experience This lady and her inside knowledge are well respected.

Sabrina Wallace / Sabrina Dawn Davis (Psinergy) - Electronic Warfare - Our Bodies are Biohacked.
https://odysee.com/@WakeUpMirror:3/swewbb:8?_ga=2.8729461.1356523320.1753223901-1387089158.1753223900
Sabrina Wallace
https://www.facebook.com/share/v/1CJfLjfgY3/?mibextid=wwXIfr
Sabrina Wallace explains the Wireless Body Area Network
https://www.facebook.com/share/v/1DK9afmP95/?mibextid=wwXIfr
Sabrina Wallace.
https://www.facebook.com/share/v/17tucmo8rs/?mibextid=wwXIfr

Sabrina Wallace
https://rumble.com/v6y0brm-nanometrology-and-environmental-monitoring.html
Sabrina Wallace
https://www.facebook.com/share/v/1CJfLjfgY3/?mibextid=wwXIfr

Psinergy
Nanometrology & Environmental Monitoring
https://rumble.com/v6y0brm-nanometrology-and-environmental-monitoring.html

Invisible weapons in action:
https://x.com/hustlebitch_/status/2010798039070622007?s=12

Dr Rima Laibow and the sudden deaths.
https://substack.com/@mitchsantell1/note/c-157240568?r=149bj4&utm_medium=ios&utm_source=notes-share-action

Nicholas Hulsher talks about damage from the COVID shots
https://rumble.com/v71dupo-top-epidemiologist-exposes-the-link-between-mrna-vaccines-and-turbo-cancers.html

Dr Deagle and early chemtrail disclosure ...
https://x.com/xphoenixdragon/status/2003624890369450346?s=46&t=nkWTOBihgJ1KldA6v7wgHQ

Old hearings on Chemtrails
https://x.com/thehealthb0t/status/1926024139665477982?s=46&t=nkWTOBihgJ1KldA6v7wgHQ.

Amazon Prime documentary (trailer)
Climate trails
https://www.instagram.com/reel/DQhxzP1AdDj/?igsh=dTJnejd6d2ZxbzZj

Interview with Blake Horowitz, lawyer on one of the geoengineering cases

https://x.com/tboo211/status/2012482148905710023?s=12

Court hearing on heavy metals from chemtrails

https://x.com/rjnol/status/1928822220333203748?s=46&t=nkWTOBihgJ1KldA6v7wgHQ

Chemtrails Timelapse

https://x.com/chemtrail101/status/1947436139792789969?s=46&t=nkWTOBihgJ1KldA6v7wgHQ

Britain's Andrew Brigden talks about chemtrails and geoengineering

https://www.facebook.com/share/v/17XYd2hQAK/?mibextid=wwXIfr

Children's Health Defense Control Is the 'Holy Grail': CHD Panel Debates Geoengineering, Earth's Future

https://childrenshealthdefense.org/defender/chd-panel-debates-geoengineering-earths-future/

Invisible weapons in action:

https://x.com/hustlebitch_/status/2010798039070622007?s=12

Dr Ed Group talks about the contents of some chemtrails
https://x.com/valerieanne1970/status/1960972361815282125?s=12

Bio engineering facts Dr Ilya Sandra Perlingieri
https://www.facebook.com/share/v/1KCE3ZFJci/?

Dane Wigington interviews Dr Allan Buckman, an trained and experienced observer of weather, plant and animal life:
https://x.com/nogps1/status/1999624437121872284?s=46&t=nkWTOBihgJ1KldA6v7wgHQ

It's more than weather control. What's in the chemtrails?
https://x.com/nogps1/status/1999993968642408510?s=46&t=nkWTOBihgJ1KldA6v7wgHQ

Chemtrails disclosure
https://x.com/conspiracyb0t/status/1999193881250795664?s=46&t=nkWTOBihgJ1KldA6v7wgHQ

Kristen Meghan, Environmental Specialist and U.S. Army whistleblower talks briefly about harmful geo-engineering
https://substack.com/@lastcall1/note/c-117792145?r=149bj4&utm_medium=ios&utm_source=notes-share-action

Geoengineering Whistleblower @KristenMeghan tells all about what 'they' are spraying in our skies here in America and around the world.

https://x.com/realericmoutsos/status/2001482981211570235?s=46&t=nkWTOBihgJ1KldA6v7wgHQ

Tucker Carlson interviews Peter A Kirby,

https://x.com/nogps1/status/2009641350476574966?s=46&t=nkWTOBihgJ1KldA6v7wgHQ

Dr Ed Group on bioengineering

https://www.facebook.com/share/r/1HA4DMuDK7/?mibextid=wwXIfr

AI talks about chemtrails ….. interesting

https://www.facebook.com/share/v/1Dr1DgwsUs/?mibextid=wwXIfr

A list of scientists who have been killed in mysterious circumstances on the verge of major breakthroughs in technology

https://x.com/iluminatibot/status/1999835182161953036?s=46&t=nkWTOBihgJ1KldA6v7wgHQ

Supplements and general detoxing

Dr Ed Group shows Patrick Gentempo around the Global Healing supplement factory

https://www.vigilantfox.com/p/who-really-owns-the-supplements-youre?utm_campaign=post&utm_medium=web

Dr Ed Group talks about the huge number of functions regulated by the liver ….

https://www.facebook.com/share/r/1BzbmLpJX3/?mibextid=wwXIfr

Ed Group talks about the importance of cleansing the liver
'A clean liver can completely reactivate your body's own self-healing mechanism.'
Dr Ed Group NP
CEO Global Healing Centre

https://youtube.com/shorts/gSFO0eY3Ilc?si=gFwyQZz-20nGtuen

Ivermectin

https://x.com/Fa21519230/status/2063392500350361992/video/1?s=46

The importance of grounding

https://x.com/tedlogan1010/status/1952329520662315125?s=46&t=nkWTOBihgJ1KldA6v7wgHQ

Better gut health using oxygen and iodine

Dr Edward Group / 766 / Dave Asprey

https://youtu.be/qDKZ0C4mRM8?si=GUOZbyOG8DJwuLe0

Dr Ken Stoller talks a little about hyperbaric oxygen and more about medical corruption.

https://rumble.com/v6slzen-questions-and-answers-on-the-health-benefits-of-hyperbaric-oxygen-therapy-w.html

Dr Eric Berg: The benefits of hyperbaric oxygen therapy.

https://youtu.be/H-8mZBkgKfQ?si=Z2rltZme6VC8LjGH

Liver cleanse

Dr Ed Group talks about the 6-day liver cleanse:

https://rumble.com/v5jime5-step-three-6-day-liver-cleanse-protocol.html

Reasons to drink structured water

https://daveasprey.com/reasons-to-drink-structured-water/

Benefits of Fulvic Acid: Dr Eric Berg:

https://youtu.be/3myDiaxX4Ts?si=6UfvPBVM5K_mTWYC

A doctor talks about the effects of artificial perfumes and scents on the body

https://youtube.com/shorts/5i4FTksm6M4?si=zv1In5i8G20aaQbm

Long article from the Midwestern Doctor on the realities of shedding: What We've Learned from a Year of Vaccine Shedding Data

https://www.midwesterndoctor.com/p/what-weve-learned-from-a-year-of?utm_source=post-email

Energy and vibration in supplements
Dr Ed Group shows us some amazing clips.

https://youtu.be/LRPgrjnh64U?si=WEV3mA4clqoZl_QX

Do Ionic Foot Baths Really Work for Detox?
with Mark Axelson and Dr. Terrance Cooper.
Myers Detox

https://rumble.com/v497fti-do-ionic-foot-baths-really-work-for-detox-with-mark-axelson-and-dr.-terranc.html

How to Strengthen your Biofield, with Sabrina Wallace, Chris Crutchfield, and Eileen McKusick

*https://youtu.be/7x3P1npQmYA?si=5SqXO8rDMoXlj5Q_*

Breathing

Dr Ed group talks about breathing energy into your body

https://youtube.com/shorts/3HQsiMQ4rfM?si=fZI3YS9FqrASVrQZ

Nebulizing Saline for RSV or Hydrogen Peroxide for Lung Ailments

https://deeprootsathome.com/nebulizing-saline-or-hydrogen-peroxide-for-lung-ailments-rsv/?fbclid=IwZnRzaANIr8NleHRuA2FlbQIxMQABHvVSoAso1Oea1PqjZtkifbE8wYSeDdnvMlkV5EISCbRP4e24Ds6EjAyUOtz5_aem_cEmgzftIJ0AgzpCzztZAEg

James Roguski: ebook 'The Truth about Food Grade Hydrogen Peroxide'

https://archive.org/details/the-truth-about-fghp_202311

EMF Radiation ☢️

https://www.facebook.com/share/v/1APNyPugVE/?

Dr Eric Berg talks about activated charcoal

https://youtu.be/lF1Cnb_VZ2g?si=pE_jNrJgRtR8Hkxp

Gut Health: Dr Sabine Hazan talks about bifida bacteria in the gut in the pre and post COVID shot era

https://www.facebook.com/share/r/1BpnXGhhb6/?mibextid=wwXIfr

What We've Learned from a Year of Covid Vaccine Shedding Data

https://x.com/midwesterndoc/status/1989717795429380117?s=46&t=nkWTOBihgJ1KldA6v7wgHQ

Dr Scott Scherr talks about hyperbaric oxygen Therapy (HBOT)

https://youtu.be/uaZNFWb9pxg?si=YwS9uldSLFya8aEY

Iodine, Selenium and Boron with Dr. Rich Olree.
An important look at foundational minerals often lacking in our soils and bodies.

https://youtu.be/H_7Ubpa4aHU?si=VZwxXf9oV61cRJ3l

Live :lood analysis

Candida and leaky gut.
Nomoresilence

https://rumble.com/v6vno45-live-blood-analysis-showing-a-leaky-gut.html

Live Blood Analysis intro
Nomoresilence

https://rumble.com/v6ybo3y-live-blood-analysis-intro.html

Ria's close ups of hydrogel, puddles and nanobots

https://www.facebook.com/reel/1379525793854099/?fs=e&mibextid=wwXIfr

Ria No More Silence: Calamari clots

https://www.facebook.com/share/r/1B15ZHN7cz/?mibextid=wwXIfr

Nanotech and calamari clots
Some of the nanotech patents

https://eccentrik.substack.com/p/we-just-hit-the-motherload

A great and concise clip on the rubbery clots by EO Nutrition, the issue and several potential answers, often with links to original studies

https://youtu.be/lyOszvJL9EU?si=nVna602xQbtqDlDS

Tom Haviland talks about the truth and the silence over rubbery clots.

https://rumble.com/v74jmd2-the-big-mig-show.html

Dr Eric Berg on what he would do if he had stage 4 cancer. Interesting ..

https://youtube.com/shorts/6aitl1Bfr1o?si=TFuTGepNfv2tVvnr

*The importance of Zeta potential (Joe Mercola and the MidWestern Doctor.)

https://articles.mercola.com/sites/articles/archive/2026/01/09/zeta-potential-vaccine-injuries-blood-sludging.aspx?cid_source=takecontrol&cid_medium=email&cid_content=art1Bttn&cid=20260209_TC&utm_source=substack&utm_medium=email

https://open.substack.com/pub/amidwesterndoctor/p/what-makes-all-vaccines-so-dangerous?utm_campaign=post&utm_medium=email

What's Really Falling From the Sky When It Snows?

https://youtu.be/1IetTEZ2RBo

Why hydrogel fuel cells are a key component in the human body

https://open.substack.com/pub/sam368/p/why-hydrogel-fuel-cells-are-a-key?r=149bj4&utm_medium=ios&shareImageVariant=overlay

Dr John Campbell with John O' Looney - White clots and sudden death

https://rumble.com/v4cj3rc-dr-john-campbell-with-john-o-looney-white-clots-and-sudden-death.html

White Clots proof
John Campbell
https://youtu.be/d2YiNVgot-A?si=bDG6gvr7xIu9Q_Pk

White clot Science
John Campbell
https://youtu.be/GEmJGuIsDkw?si=J-TJxx0xC9_0TIr4

Bloodstream Code Red: The Amyloid Clots in COVID's Wake That Nobody's Discussing
Bloodstream Code Red: The Amyloid Clots in COVID's Wake That Nobody's Discussing - Vejon Health

Lee Merritt MD interviews Maria Crisler on hydrogel, frequency, parasites and hope.
The Medical Rebel
https://rumble.com/v5anlgp-dr-lee-merritt-the-medical-rebel-maria-crisler-on-hydrogel-frequency-and-ho.html

Maria Zee talks to Ana Milhacea.
A dramatic interview spelling out some dark possibilities of the nanotech in our blood.
https://cairnsnews.org/2025/08/15/dr-ana-mihalcea-describes-how-nanobots-have-taken-over-vaxxed-and-un-vaxxed-bodies/

Ana Milhacea on the Iron Will podcast

https://anamihalceamdphd.substack.com/p/iron-will-podcast-we-are-all-infected?r=149bj4&utm_medium=ios&utm_campaign=audio-player

A spectacular and disturbing interview: Dr Ana Milhacea talks to a very experienced nurse, doctor and microscopist of 30 years: Dr Sandy Corlett ND, ThD, DDiv, DCC, PScD.
(two links for the same clip.)

https://rumble.com/v4t4lb2-nanotechnology-warfare-against-humanity-seen-in-live-blood-conversation-wit.html

https://open.substack.com/pub/anamihalceamdphd/p/nanotechnology-warfare-against-humanity?r=149bj4&utm_medium=ios

Live blood analysis training and slides. Nomoresilence gives us a brief look at bright field and dark field slides.

https://rumble.com/v5e4999-live-blood-analysis-training-and-slides.html

Rianomoresilence:
Junctions in nano-filaments on different continents

https://www.facebook.com/share/v/1AVLZc3PkQ/?mibextid=wwXIfr

Details of the components of some nanotechnology
Dr Ed Group talks about components of the nanotechnology
https://x.com/valerieanne1970/status/19609723618152821

25?s=46&t=nkWTOBihgJ1KldA6v7wgHQ
A Great overview of the nanotech by Unhackable Animal.
https://unhackableanimal.substack.com/p/video-nanotech-based-contamination?r=149bj4&utm_medium=ios&utm_campaign=audio-player

Dr David Nixon
Journal of Bionanotechnocracy
Volume 1, Issue 1 - April 2025.
Active Microscale Construction in Pfizer Comirnaty: Investigating Complex Self-Assembling Structures
Drdavidnixon.com

Dr David Nixon and nanotechnology in biological systems (bodies)
https://open.substack.com/pub/davidnixon/p/the-psyop-that-wasnt-a-response-to?r=149bj4&utm_medium=ios

Dr Ed Group talks to Jim Grapek and Charles Frohman.
https://open.substack.com/pub/yourfreedomhub/p/detoxing-from-the-clot-shot-and-shedding?r=149bj4&utm_medium=

Ana Milhacea spells out what is happening in the blood
Self Assembly Of A Mesogen Microchip In COVID19 Unvaccinated Blood and Microrobots Building a Clot:
Ana Mihalcea, MD, PHD, Nov 2025
https://open.substack.com/pub/anamihalceamdphd/p/self-assembly-of-a-mesogen-microchip?r=149bj4&utm_medium=ios

Dr Ed Group on nanotechnology
https://x.com/xphoenixdragon/status/1958848275932410363?s=46&t=nkWTOBihgJ1KldA6v7wgHQhttps://youtu.be/WP1yPCLJ6_s?si=Hu8TolkwTZjgdcEK

Red Alert. It's in our blood
Ana Milhacea
https://open.substack.com/pub/anamihalceamdphd/p/interview-on-sgt-report-red-alert?r=149bj4&utm_medium=ios

Ana Milhacea
Antidote for shedding
https://rumble.com/v5okmy5-the-antidote-for-shedding-vax-injury-and-long-covid.html

A great conversation as microbiologist Maria Crisler talks to Matt Skow and Edward Szall
The Agenda: Died suddenly
https://rumble.com/v6veekj-the-shots-corrupted-our-blood-guest-maria-crisler.html

Tom Haviland talks about the truth and the silence over rubbery clots.
https://rumble.com/v74jmd2-the-big-mig-show.html

Smart Dust is already everywhere …
Energy Reporters: a slightly different aspect of what we face.
https://www.energy-reporters.com/news/smart-dust-is-already-everywhere-microscopic-spy-sensors-track-your-location-while-tech-companies-hide-the-surveillance-revolution-forever/

All 12 Solfeggio frequencies. Dr Ed Group
https://youtu.be/N3DS3cU9To0?si=G1luV4jTsYODsmSw

Global Healing: six secrets to total body detox.
https://globalhealinginstitute.org/dr-groups-6-secrets-to-total-body-detox/?uid=28&oid=16&affid=2

Global healing on parasites: a paid course:
https://globalhealinginstitute.org/why-everyone-needs-a-parasite-cleanse/?uid=22&oid=16&affid=2

Dr Henry Ealy talks about sweating out chemtrail toxins

https://www.facebook.com/share/v/17ncUz2qF7/?mibextid=wwXIfr

Scientist and inventor Filipe Reitz speaks to Ana Milhacea about thermography for clots and blockages in veins and arteries. July 2024

https://rumble.com/v57gxql-computerized-thermography-and-live-blood-analysis-conversation-with-felipe-.html

Blue tooth MAC address phenomenon from Covid 19 shots. Conversation with Dr Pedro Chavez from COMUSAV, Truth, Light and Spirit episode 30.

https://anamihalceamdphd.substack.com/p/blue-tooth-mac-address-phenomenon?r=149bj4&utm_medium=ios&utm_campaign=audio-player

Components of the nanotechnology

https://x.com/valerieanne1970/status/1960972361815282125?s=46&t=nkWTOBihgJ1KldA6v7wgHQ

Cymatics demonstrated: frequency in action

https://youtu.be/Pmsfuj1Rk9c?si=6ssZx4DS_Sh60Yih

Other blood contamination?
Greg Reese in a brief clip on invisible glowing markers under the skin.

https://substack.com/@mtcali70/note/c-166438837?r=149bj4&utm_medium=ios&utm_source=notes-share-action

Major Tom Haviland, John O'Looney and Richard Hirschman talk to Maria Zee about rubbery clots. Zeemedia

https://rumble.com/v58wy85-major-haviland-r.-hircshman-john-olooney-white-rubbery-clots-government-ign.html

Maria Zee talks to Nicholas Hulscher from the McCullough Foundation about Amyloid clots. It's good to know that the McCullough Foundation is paying attention to this.

https://www.instagram.com/reel/DRdyZ3vDKn7/?igsh=MWZzMncwN3V3NW1pbQ==

Documenting Genocide.
The vax amyloid clots syndrome. The SGT Report with Dr Todd Callender, Australian Journalists Wayne Crouch and Lisa Johnston, Richard Hirschman, retired Major Tom Haviland, retired organic chemist, Greg Harrison. Dr Bill Lionberger, Dr Sherri Tenpenny, Dr Rima Laibow. (Maybe copy this clip and paste it into DuckDuckGo for best results)

https://www.bitchute.com/video/8oTqkjmpJQfo/

The Reese Report:
Brief clip about nano-filaments hydro gel and self assembling nano-bots.
https://rumble.com/v4u39su-self-replicating-nanobots-found-in-both-the-vaxxed-and-unvaxxed.html

Greg Reese of the Reese report speaks to (retired) Major Tom Haviland and Greg Harrison about rubbery clots.
https://gregreese.substack.com/p/clot-shot-science-with-thomas-haviland?r=149bj4&utm_medium=ios&utm_campaign=audio-player

A brief description of this research by Greg Reese
https://gregreese.substack.com/p/the-nefarious-science-behind-the?r=149bj4&utm_medium=ios&utm_campaign=audio-player

EDTA

An important clip of EDTA and vitamin C breaking down rubbery clots. nomoresilence
https://rumble.com/v6toaj3-edta-and-vit-c-breaking-down-rubbery-clots.html

Dr Ana Milhacea talks to Dr Michael Roth about the many benefits of EDTA.

Humanity United Now

https://rumble.com/v1wpt6e-edta-detoxification-for-metals-graphene-and-hydrogel.html

E:OO

EBOO (extra corporeal blood oxygenation and ozonation therapy) in action at Auckland clinic

https://www.instagram.com/reel/DNRpdEfyaga/?igsh=NmxrbWdkcTZ1ZjE3

Tiny clip of a long clot being pulled out of an EBOO (extra corporeal blood oxygenation and ozonation therapy) line.

https://www.instagram.com/reel/DQ4yovYktzk/?igsh=MXUybDQ0eWI4ZGI2OQ==

Cancer

The Gerson institute.
Founded by Charlotte Gerson, daughter of Dr Max Gerson.

https://gerson.org/about-us/

Charlotte Gerson on cancer

https://rumble.com/v4sbrnn-charlotte-gerson-what-is-cancer-gerson-institute-archives.html

Hoxey Bio Medical Centre

https://www.hoxseybiomedical.com/

Dr Peter Glidden on cancer and chemotherapy

https://rumble.com/v2sf81w-dr.-peter-glidden-on-cancer-treatment.html

Dr Ed Group talks about parasites and healing the gut.

https://youtube.com/shorts/Z4c56IiT3As?si=2PnKBw7-djjXPKmp

The 100% truth about cancer and our sick system: SGT Report talks to John Richardson from Richardson Nutritional Center.

https://rumble.com/v4u6zxe-the-100-truth-about-cancer-and-our-sick-system-john-richardson.html

Andreas Moritz explains what cancer is doing in the body. It gives clarity on why these changes are needed:
Cancer is Not Trying to Kill You, It is Trying to Save You:

https://youtu.be/r18OHoT5Q7o?si=3kO-63M4xlqRuwKp

What chemo can do …

https://x.com/xx17965797n/status/1890345917716254981?s=46&t=nkWTOBihgJ1KldA6v7wgHQ

A Cancer Surgeon talks about cancer and Ivermectin
https://rumble.com/v6p6sgx-cancer-surgeon-talks-about-ivermectin.html

Nicholas Hulsher talks about damage from the COVID shots
https://rumble.com/v71dupo-top-epidemiologist-exposes-the-link-between-mrna-vaccines-and-turbo-cancers.html

Dr John Campbell and Dr William Makis discuss turbo cancers and repurposed drugs. A fascinating talk.
https://rumble.com/v6qm4io-dr.-campbell-and-dr.-makis-discuss-turbo-cancers-and-repurposed-drugs.html
BREAKING: Largest Human Cancer Study of Ivermectin + Mebendazole.

PEER-REVIEWED and PUBLISHED in a Major Cancer Journal.

84.4% of cancer patients taking ivermectin + mebendazole for 6 months reported either CANCER DISAPPEARANCE, TUMOR REGRESSION, or CANCER STABILIZATION.
https://open.substack.com/pub/petermcculloughmd/p/breaking-largest-human-cancer-study?r=149bj4&utm_medium=ios

Can ai tell you how to cure brain cancer naturally?
You be the judge. Some very good suggestions here.
Draw your own conclusions…
https://www.instagram.com/reel/DNAcuxUIEAJ/?igsh=MXJoNHdjMmZ4OXNzYQ==

One Answer to Cancer
Elaine Hollingsworth
https://youtu.be/MR3oUleXieM?si=Nw7ePNum-jrlIX7u

This is an excellent, genuine and simple presentation: Scott Bennett, Healing Cancer with Indian Black Salve
https://youtu.be/MR3oUleXieM?si=cOFWL7slsyDy5GAx

Dr William Makis MD,
https://makismd.substack.com/p/exclusive-interview-maria-zee-on?r=149bj4&utm_mediu

Interview with Dr. William Makis on Using IVERMECTIN and FENBENDAZOLE to Treat/Cure Cancer
https://rumble.com/v5sih0w-dr-william-makis-ivermectin.html

Dr William Makis talks briefly about ivermectin
https://x.com/realfletch17/status/1918653776593821879?s=46&t=nkWTOBihgJ1KldA6v7wgHQ

Dr Eric Berg is a great resource on general health and medical issues:
Cancer dies when you do this
https://youtu.be/f9PL6o4OLNw?si=P39i9hiZMomWGChB

Dr Berg's Five diet strategies for cancer care:
This is an important PDF.
https://drbrg.co/4om43oQ

Dr. Lee Merritt – SHOCK Discovery – Parasites: Cancer & Turbo Cancer Breakthrough. Zeemedia
https://rumble.com/v5vqgah-dr.-lee-merritt-shock-discovery-parasites-cancer-and-turbo-cancer-breakthro.html

Dr Lee Merritt.com, the Medical Rebel
There is a detailed parasite removal protocol you can print off in PDF from her website
https://drleemerritt.com/

Dr. Merritt and Attorney Todd Calendar on the Enemy within The Medical Rebel. This is a fascinating and wide ranging discussion from 2023
https://rumble.com/v45696i-dr.-merritt-and-attorney-todd-calendar-on-the-enemy-within.html

Studying Otto Warburg's hypothesis over 70 years on
We've Been Fighting Cancer the Wrong Way — Until Now
https://youtu.be/Pl5Nt3WrV5E

Dr Thomas Seyfried: New study Confirms that cancer cells ferment Glutamine.
https://youtu.be/KjdAtauO2cA?si=9sZ9TMUUVwUXtBS5

Talking cancer with Professor Thomas N Seyfried
https://youtu.be/KjdAtauO2cA

Trio infernal against Cancer
Curing cancer
Dr Andreas Kalcker
https://open.substack.com/pub/drkalcker/p/trio-infernal-against-cancer?r=149bj4&utm_medium=ios

Dr Lee Merritt talks about parasites:
Parasites--a New Paradigm
the Medical Rebel
https://rumble.com/v1owcgh-parasites-a-new-paradigm.html

Dr William Makis MD,
https://makismd.substack.com/p/exclusive-interview-maria-zee-on?r=149bj4&utm_medium=ios&utm_campaign=audio-player

Sound frequency kills cancer cells.
This technology appears to be very like that developed by Royal Raymond Rife over 80 years ago
https://www.facebook.com/share/r/1DC9trc6zV/?mibextid=wwXIfr

Histotripsy is in essence a continuation of Rife's work and destroys cancer cells using frequency. Interesting that the presenter is Sara Rothschild of the Life Raft Group …
I haven't listened to this one so draw your own conclusions.

Histotripsy Demystified: Truths & Misconceptions Explained - Expert panel
https://youtu.be/5JNarCfHomM?si=GYqs2RzXotVHUiJI

Dr Deitrich Klinghardt from the Klinghardt Institute and the cocktail of frequency, aluminium and glyphosate we live in …
https://x.com/JohnFkennedy324/status/2063552655700398428/video/1?s=46

Dr. Lee Merritt – SHOCK Discovery – Parasites: Cancer & Turbo Cancer Breakthrough. ZeeeMedia
https://rumble.com/v5vqgah-dr.-lee-merritt-shock-discovery-parasites-cancer-and-turbo-cancer-breakthro.html

Dr Lee Merritt

Cancer and parasites

Dangerous Dames I Ep.17: ViroLIEgy & The Cancer/Parasite Connection & More!

https://rumble.com/v4bnmo2-dangerous-dames-ep.17-viroliegy-and-the-cancerparasite-connection-and-more.html

Venoms and nicotine

Short clip on nicotine's action in the body

https://www.facebook.com/share/r/16b4Ge5H9Y/?mibextid=wwXIfr

Dr Bryan Ardis talks about snake venoms as the source of covid

https://rumble.com/v1sd6bi-australiaone-update.-interview-with-dr-bryan-ardis-and-riccardo-bosi.html

Maria Crisler talks to Brian Ardis about snake venoms

https://rumble.com/v6revns-the-ultimate-parasite-cleanse-including-synthetic.html

:io engineering

Long article from the Midwestern Doctor on the realities of shedding: What We've Learned from a Year of Vaccine Shedding Data

https://www.midwesterndoctor.com/p/what-weve-learned-from-a-year-of?utm_source=post-email

Dr Paul Marik talks about spike protein harms:

https://substack.com/@stopthoseshots/note/c-183666602?r=149bj4&utm_medium=ios

Methylene-blue

I think these articles and clips are balanced and informative.

The Real Health Podcast by the Riordan Clinic: The Anti-oxidant power of methylene-blue with Dr Ron Hunninghake and Dr Thomas Levy.

https://youtu.be/lo1oTJDUXtY?si=OxY6m9jaG-PxTxci

The Real Health Podcast by the Riordan Clinic: A second look at methylene-blue with Dr Ron Hunninghake and Dr Thomas Levy.

https://youtu.be/lq7MWWPfSTY?si=QL1mGaJtlAMbFEbc

Exploring the Health benefits of methylene-blue with Dr Thomas Levy

https://youtu.be/2GYdo1-5ZUU?si=8n_8JCwAbiCUVwB9

Detailed talk on methylene-blue
Dr John Lieurance

https://youtu.be/TR-jyx6CFss?si=wz6WqYIFk-szSSK9

Dr Paul Anderson, integrative and naturopathic doctor speaks about methylene-blue:
Everything you need to know about Methylene Blue

https://youtu.be/bfPByasoJTw?si=51rjonw4dZj0dzMY

Give me 36 minutes. I'll explain everything about methylene-blue … Dr Paul Anderson ND (I think this clip is particularly detailed and balanced).

https://youtu.be/AJOk_0ggxm4?si=QEd2gvMatzewb1yl

A brief summary of methylene-blue

https://x.com/jasper_truth/status/1891896153471340691?s=46&t=nkWTOBihgJ1KldA6v7wgHQ

Dr Brandon Crawford speaks about methylene-blue

https://youtu.be/-3gvKoRTmTY?si=NbADJZGr_MuAd9G5

Jonas Kuehne on the science and benefits of methylene-blue.

https://youtu.be/x7PPLiueLWs?si=Z1iWvblT2yiiLxjJ

Dosing and safety of methylene-blue.
Jonas Kuehne
https://youtu.be/WNqTUyLLIdI?si=bFBjHYfsRpq7L0PA

History, science and benefits of methylene-blue
https://globalhealinginstitute.org/healinglibrary/the-history-science-and-benefits-of-methylene-blue/

The incredible impacts of Methylene Blue (Research backed)
https://youtu.be/jXijx_VICRI?si=7o80SICtzVMaTG7Q

Dr Jonas Kuehne talks about the 'BLUE BRAIN' FEAR-MONGERING and the benefits of methylene-blue
https://youtube.com/shorts/MW11E-2qIl8?si=hlLL9Ln3mBQ_Pnkq

Dr Scott Scherr answers questions about methylene-blue
Part 1
https://youtu.be/qdN3q8MFJIM?si=wNfkUZ36On2wVvAL
Part 2
https://youtu.be/XcBwDwkjhMI?si=upG0EoVH6yID4wGy

Dr Scott Sherr from Troscriptions addresses some of the concerns raised by Paul Saladino's recent video on methylene blue (link below). This response clarifies key misunderstandings around dosage, serotonin syndrome, mitochondrial function, and synthetic ingredients.
https://youtu.be/GCUgSX4rMtM

Dr Scott Scherr: methylene-blue and sperm health.
https://youtube.com/shorts/SXSyg2b7PVY?si=4xAjetMSbi6CkUkR

Dr Scherr talks about Troscriptions methylene-blue testing
https://youtube.com/shorts/n0Vi25GmFLo?si=hlwRNpnxhvqhoCBU

Ana Milhacea recommends methylene-blue to prevent the spread of nanoparticles. This is a more scientific starter point which would benefit from more investigation
https://open.substack.com/pub/anamihalceamdphd/p/methylene-blue-inhibits-nano-and?r=149bj4&utm_medium=ios

Methylene Blue
Miracle Molecule or Psyop?
Alyce Harms
https://drive.google.com/file/d/1xUyUJ4RoNPiqKCFxqJ61p8lMicDmlJne/view

Important and detailed description of methylene-blue
https://metabolichealth.com/methylene-blue-history-uses-and-benefits/

You'll find this study on the Pubmed website by keying in the PMID number. This is a very important study at this time because our blood may be compromised and may lead to issues like sepsis

Paul Marik, MBBCh

Sepsis becomes more likely as the blood loses its energy and oxygen.

Hydrocortisone, Vitamin C, and Thiamine for the Treatment of Severe Sepsis and Septic Shock: A Retrospective Before-After Study. PMID 27940189.

The ELFET/Tri-Vortex green laser technology draws on the information embedded in sacred geometry.

Crop circles

https://x.com/redpilldispensr/status/1993266783344603529?s=46&t=nkWTOBihgJ1KldA6v7wgHQ

Dr Lee Merritt

Cancer and parasites

Dangerous Dames I Ep.17: ViroLIEgy & The Cancer/Parasite Connection & More!

https://rumble.com/v4bnmo2-dangerous-dames-ep.17-viroliegy-and-the-cancerparasite-connection-and-more.html

If this doesn't send us running for the parasite cleanses, nothing will. A coroner speaks:

https://x.com/jasielcth/status/2040444718409208139?s=46&t=nkWTOBihgJ1KldA6v7wgHQ

A small clip on the importance of deworming parasites:

https://x.com/thehealthb0t/status/2040566481948422636?s=46&t=nkWTOBihgJ1KldA6v7wgHQ

Cancer - a Parasitical infection. Video proof

https://rumble.com/v2vyiu8-video-proof-cancer-is-caused-by-parasites.html

Graphene Oxide in dental anaesthetics

Removing or moving out of the way? An interesting clip for dentists and anyone giving anaesthetics. I really respect this narrator, but I have also heard from aware dentists and experienced microscopists that this doesn't work, not least because graphene is carbon and not magnetic.

I have included this clip because people sometimes refer to it. I do not believe this works. Being practical, I also don't believe that you could persuade your dentist to do it.

So far, only the Elfet Tri-Vortex chamber disrupts the self-assembly ability of the nano-filaments, rendering them much less harmful. Draw your own conclusions

https://www.facebook.com/share/r/14wZJVpsPN/?mibextid=UalRPS

Nanotechnology: The Future of Conservative Dentistry and Endodontics @DentalAddaDrSwarneet. There is a huge amount of new information on a revolutionary new technology in this short clip, presented as if it is both tested and safe. (After 16 years in the vaccine truth space, I question both these assumptions.)

https://youtu.be/_XG2wHpWQtI?si=7N6vtGwj48EpthQV

Dr William Makis talks about persecution and Ivermectin

https://www.facebook.com/share/r/1BbupvEw9n/?mibextid=wwXIfr

Steve Ross PhD talks about Royal Raymond Rife and his microscopes.

The suppressed cure. How big Pharma and government buried Rife's disease-killing breakthroughs.

https://rumble.com/v59xr7h-the-suppressed-cure-how-big-pharma-and-government-buried-rifes-disease-kill.html

Royal Raymond Rife and the resurrection of resonance. (copy and paste the link to access this interesting piece. Note that Rife himself uses the word virus when describing what he was seeing.)

https://rumble.com/v6tcw2v-royal-rife-and-the-resurrection-of-resonance-reclaim-the-terrain-episode-2.html

Royal Rife BX Virus Laboratory Research, with specific detail.

https://youtu.be/x9eQiFdK19Q?si=tkbHsLuGr6ygalqV

Tony Pantalleresco: website

https://powerofthepulse.com/tony/nano-basics/

Tony Pantalleresco original video - making the anti-nano buckets

https://rumble.com/v4e3koc-how-to-building-the-anti-nano-bucket-tony-pantalleresco.html

A more detailed description of how to make the nano bucket.

https://youtu.be/v7pJ3Lhdx_A?si=zY_JR2VLd7RhUCtx

Anti Nano bucket

https://rumble.com/vswpkv-anti-nano-devices-trainingwebinar.-what-you-need-to-know-to-select-the-corr.html

Anti nano larger bucket
More refined

https://youtu.be/NdKXbrmXu4k?si=VnU7jrL6KntfFbiR

Tony Pantalleresco
Anti nano triangle

https://rumble.com/v578gkl-anti-nano-triangle-tony-pantalleresco-backup.html

Daisy Hinesley - Update to "Tony Pantalleresco's AntiNano Bucket Works!" (Originally Posted: November 11, 2024)
https://open.substack.com/pub/nanostructuresinus/p/update-to-tony-pantallerescos-antinano?r=149bj4&utm_medium=ios&shareImageVariant=overlay

Susanne Maher talks to Tony Pantalleresco and Bryan 396 about Morgellons and nanotechnology
https://rumble.com/v6q6gdq-morgellons-bryan396-tony-pantalleresco-and-suzanne-maher-2017.html

Maria Crisler presents on Nanotechnology and human beings
https://dhughes.substack.com/p/presentation-by-maria-crisler-april?r=149bj4&utm_medium=ios&utm_campaign=audio-player

Blue tooth MAC address phenomenon from Covid 19 shots. Conversation with Dr Pedro Chavez from COMUSAV, Truth, Light and Spirit episode 30.
https://anamihalceamdphd.substack.com/p/blue-tooth-mac-address-phenomenon?r=149bj4&utm_medium=ios&utm_campaign=audio-player

Components of the nanotechnology

https://x.com/valerieanne1970/status/1960972361815282125?s=46&t=nkWTOBihgJ1KldA6v7wgHQ

Naturecure Academy

https://www.livebloodanalysistraining.com/

I like the clear way the Naturecure Academy presents its certified courses and the specials for appropriate quality dark field microscopes and monitor- linked cameras.

https://naturecure-academy.myshopify.com/

Live Blood on Line

Information on live blood analysis, the equipment and training needed.

https://livebloodonline.com

Long list of free energy inventors found dead in mysterious circumstances

https://x.com/xx17965797n/status/1937474725610983682?s=46&t=nkWTOBihgJ1KldA6v7wgHQ

Delivering truth with wit as ever, Katie Hopkins sums up many people's feelings on the medical industry perfectly.

The end of the God delusion.

https://www.facebook.com/share/r/1L7ktdpCKL/?mibextid=wwXlfr

Mistakes were not made.

An Anthem for Justice

By Margaret Anna Alice

Read by Dr Tess Lawrie

https://youtu.be/ueUXNL-A3Zg

Made in the USA
Las Vegas, NV
04 November 2026

57437106R00240